T0222985

# EMQs for the MRCOG Part 2:
## The Essential Guide

# EMQs for the MRCOG Part 2:
## The Essential Guide

**Andrea Pilkington, MRCOG, PG Dip Med Ed**
*Trainee in Obstetrics and Gynaecology, North West Deanery, UK*

**Amitabha Majumdar, MRCOG**
*Consultant in Obstetrics and Gynaecology,*
*University Hospital South Manchester, UK*

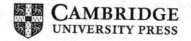
CAMBRIDGE
UNIVERSITY PRESS

# CAMBRIDGE
## UNIVERSITY PRESS

University Printing House, Cambridge CB2 8BS, United Kingdom

Cambridge University Press is part of the University of Cambridge.

It furthers the University's mission by disseminating knowledge in the pursuit of
education, learning and research at the highest international levels of excellence.

www.cambridge.org
Information on this title: www.cambridge.org/9781107687103

First published 2015

*A catalogue record for this publication is available from the British Library*

*Library of Congress Cataloguing in Publication data*
Pilkington, Andrea, author.
EMQs for the MRCOG Part 2 : the essential guide / Andrea Pilkington,
Amitabha Majumdar.
    p. ; cm.
Includes bibliographical references and index.
ISBN 978-1-107-68710-3 (Paperback)
I. Majumdar, Amitabha, author.  II. Title.
[DNLM:  1. Obstetrics–Great Britain–Examination Questions.  2. Gynecology–
Great Britain–Examination Questions.   WQ 18.2]
RG111
618.076–dc23   2014022410

ISBN 978-1-107-68710-3 Paperback

. . . . . . . . . . . . . . . . . . . . . . . . . . . . . . . . . . . . . . . . . . . . . . . . . . . . . . . . . . . . . . . . . . . . . . . . . . . . . . . . . . . . . . . . . . . . . . . . . . . . . . . . .

Dedicated to our families, Richard and William, and Chandrima and Anudarshi, for their support and patience whilst we have been writing!

# CONTENTS

# ACKNOWLEDGEMENTS

Our thanks go to those who have helped review and edit our questions and provided us with invaluable constructive feedback – Mr G Okunoye, Dr S Loveridge, Dr C Langley, Dr K Gossage, and all those who have helped who wish to remain nameless!

# PREFACE

This exciting new book of extended matching questions is written for candidates taking the MRCOG Part 2 examination.

The book contains 150 EMQs, together with answers that have full detailed explanations and references for further reading to enhance knowledge and understanding, unlike many other books on the market. A handy hints and tips section on passing the exam is also included to improve candidates' chances of exam success!

*EMQs for the MRCOG Part 2: The Essential Guide* is an invaluable study aid to help pass the EMQ component of the MRCOG Part 2!

# Introduction: How to answer EMQs for the MRCOG Part 2 and general revision hints and tips

## Know your stuff!: read all relevant guidelines and *The Obstetrician and Gynaecologist*

Many of the EMQs are based upon up-to-date guidelines used by the Royal College of Obstetricians and Gynaecologists, or those used by obstetricians and gynaecologists in the UK such as NICE (National Institute for Health and Care Excellence) and the FSRH (Faculty of Sexual and Reproductive Healthcare). You will find references to these guidelines in the answers for each question in this book.

Answer each question just as the guideline suggests or states. It may be that there is more than one good answer to a question, but the most appropriate will usually be the one that relates to a guideline.

## Cover over the options list to avoid getting distracted

If your knowledge is up-to-date and accurate, then you will most likely know the answer to a question once you have read it. Therefore, looking at the option list first will only distract you and may lead you to doubt yourself.

A better strategy is to read the question (more than once) with the list of options covered up and then look for your answer within the list. If your answer is not there (!), then re-read the question to see what subtlety you may have missed.

## Don't rush in with your first answer: there may be a better one!

Sometimes, there may be two similar answers – only one of which is the correct and most appropriate answer. Therefore, ensure that you have read the full list of options before answering the question.

## Use your clinical time wisely

Every patient you see in clinic or whilst on call you can treat as a potential EMQ or other style of exam question. For example, if you see a patient with polycystic ovarian syndrome in clinic, ask yourself, 'What does it state in the guideline about this condition?' Then, read the guideline either before or after you have seen the patient to cement the information in your head.

## Practice, practice, practice!

Practice makes perfect, and this is certainly true with EMQs. Make use of the various books available (including this one!). Some may not necessarily be in the exact style of the exam, but will allow you to test your revision and acquired knowledge!

Ask others to test you, including at work when you have a spare minute; perhaps on nights, so that every part of your day can be used for revision.

## Work in revision groups

Revision for an exam can be a lonely process. Working in groups for at least part of your revision time can make it more enjoyable (if there can be such a thing!) and allow you to gain knowledge from each other which may just stick.

# OBSTETRICS

# RHESUS D PROPHYLAXIS

## Options

A   500 IU anti-D
B   Kleihauer and 500 IU anti-D
C   250 IU anti-D
D   Kleihauer and 250 IU anti-D
E   No anti-D required
F   Anti-D at 6-weekly intervals
G   Large dose (2500 or 5000 IU) anti-D required
H   Give RAADP (routine antenatal Anti-D prophylaxis)
I   Check antibody screen and give RAADP
J   Check antibody screen at booking and at 28 weeks

## What would be the most appropriate management in each scenario?

1   A 28-year-old RhD-negative woman in her first pregnancy undergoes a fetal loss at 21 weeks of gestation.
2   A 30-year-old RhD-negative woman has a threatened miscarriage at 14 weeks of gestation in her first pregnancy and anti-D prophylaxis is administered. Bleeding continues three days later but then stops, and once again one week later.
3   A 39-year-old RhD-negative woman in her third pregnancy (non-sensitised) wishes to be sterilised after birth and declines RAADP.
4   A RhD-negative woman receives 30 mls of a blood transfusion, before discovering that she has been given RhD-positive blood.

# CHICKENPOX IN PREGNANCY

## Options

A   Test for VZV (varicella zoster virus) immunity
B   Administer VZIG (varicella zoster immunoglobulin) as soon as possible
C   No risk, therefore nil required
D   Refer to Fetal Medicine Unit for fetal testing
E   Administer VZIG in the next 48 hours
F   Administer VZIG and manage as potentially infectious from 8–28 days after administration
G   Administer VZIG and manage as potentially infectious from 8–21 days after administration
H   Administer VZIG and monitor for 28 days after administration
I    Oral acyclovir
J    Intravenous acyclovir

## What would be the most appropriate management in each scenario?

5   A pregnant woman at 22 weeks of gestation is admitted to the antenatal ward with an antepartum haemorrhage. Whilst an inpatient on a ward, she has contact with a child who has a chickenpox rash all over her body and the vesicles have not crusted over. Testing of the woman reveals she is non-immune to VZV.

6   A pregnant woman at 39 weeks of gestation develops shingles following contact with a child with chickenpox. She has a normal delivery three days later of a baby boy weighing 3695 g. What is the most appropriate management for the neonate?

7   A woman delivers a baby girl at 40 weeks and develops a chickenpox rash three days post delivery. What is the most appropriate management for the neonate?

# REDUCING THE RISK OF THROMBOEMBOLISM

## Options

A   Antenatal high-dose, low-molecular-weight heparin (LMWH)
B   Antenatal LMWH and six weeks postnatal LMWH
C   Antenatal high-dose LMWH and six weeks postnatal LMWH; involve expert haematologist in care
D   Antenatal high-dose LMWH and six weeks postnatal LMWH
E   Unfractionated heparin
F   Warfarin
G   Six weeks postnatal LMWH
H   Seven days postnatal LMWH
I   Antenatal high-dose LMWH and seven days postnatal LMWH

## What would be the most appropriate management in each scenario?

8   A 32-year-old woman is seen for booking in early pregnancy. She has a family history of thrombophilia and testing reveals anti-thrombin 3 deficiency.

9   A 33-year-old woman is seen for booking in her second pregnancy with a history of a DVT at 20 weeks in her first pregnancy. Previous screening has indicated no known inherited thrombophilia.

10  A 28-year-old woman with a BMI of 40 presents at 12 weeks of gestation for booking in her first pregnancy. She smokes 20 cigarettes per day.

# THE ACUTE MANAGEMENT OF THROMBOSIS AND EMBOLISM

## Options

A   Chest X-ray
B   Full blood count
C   D-dimer
D   Renal and hepatic function test
E   CTPA (computed tomography pulmonary angiogram)
F   V-Q scan (ventilation-perfusion lung scan)
G   Bilateral lower-limb Doppler
H   Anti-Xa level
I   Spirometry
J   Lower-limb Doppler on the suspected side

## What would be the most appropriate investigation in each scenario?

11   A 25-year-old woman who is 30 weeks pregnant presents with shortness of breath, chest pain and reduced oxygen saturations. You suspect a pulmonary embolism, but the chest X-ray is normal. What would be your next line investigation?

12   A 25-year-old woman who is 28 weeks pregnant is being treated for a confirmed deep vein thrombosis and weighs 95 kg. This is her second deep vein thrombosis in the last five years. The haematologist requests an investigation on this patient.

# HYPERTENSION IN PREGNANCY

## Options

A    Do not admit patient to hospital or treat hypertension; no indication for blood tests, but monitor blood pressure weekly.

B    Do not admit patient to hospital or treat hypertension, but take blood tests and monitor blood pressure twice per week.

C    Admit patient to hospital, treat hypertension with oral anti-hypertensives, consider steroids and early delivery.

D    Admit patient to hospital, treat hypertension with IV anti-hypertensives, take blood pressure at least four times per day and take a quantificative protein test.

E    Admit patient to hospital, treat hypertension with oral anti-hypertensives, take blood pressure at least four times per day and take a quantificative protein test.

F    Admit patient to hospital, treat hypertension with alternate including IV anti-hypertensives, take blood pressure at least four times per day and take a quantificative protein test. Consider the administration of steroids, discuss with consultant obstetrician, neonatal and anaesthetic staff with regards to delivery.

G    Do not admit patient to hospital, treat hypertension with oral anti-hypertensives, take blood pressure at least twice per week, take blood tests.

H    Do not admit patient to hospital, treat hypertension with oral anti-hypertensives, take blood pressure at least twice per week, no need for blood tests.

## What would be the most appropriate management in each scenario?

13    A 40-year-old woman presents at 32 weeks of gestation in her first pregnancy with a blood pressure of 143/90 mmHg. Blood pressure at the beginning of her pregnancy was 100/60 mmHg. Quantitative testing

indicated no proteinuria. She feels well, with no headaches or visual disturbance.

14  A 30-year-old woman presents at 34 weeks of gestation in her first pregnancy with a blood pressure of 152/103 (blood pressure at the beginning of pregnancy – 130/60) with significant proteinuria on urinalysis.

15  A 27-year-old woman presents at 28 weeks of gestation in her second pregnancy with a blood pressure of 152/105 (blood pressure at the beginning of pregnancy – 132/58), but with no evidence of proteinuria on urinalysis. She is commenced on oral labetalol and is sent home from the triage department to return in a week for a repeat blood pressure monitoring. At this time, she returns and her blood pressure has increased to 167/115 mmHg, with significant proteinuria on urinalysis. She has a frontal headache and describes spots in front of her eyes.

# THE DIAGNOSIS AND TREATMENT OF MALARIA IN PREGNANCY

## Options

A   Allow home with chloroquine 300 mg orally, weekly until delivery and anti-emetics, ensure a plan has been formulated with the multi-disciplinary team for management of recurrence and future antenatal care/delivery.

B   Admit to hospital, administer oral quinine 600 mg 8-hourly and oral clindamycin 450 mg 8-hourly for seven days, administer anti-emetics and make a plan with the multi-disciplinary team for management of recurrence and future antenatal care/delivery.

C   Allow home with oral primaquine 15 mg single daily dose for 14 days and anti-emetics, ensure a plan has been formulated with the multi-disciplinary team for management of recurrence and future antenatal care/delivery.

D   Admit to hospital, administer primaquine 45–60 mg orally once a week for eight weeks and anti-emetics, ensure a plan has been formulated with the multi-disciplinary team for management of recurrence and future antenatal care/delivery.

E   Admit to Intensive Care Unit and administer artesunate IV 2.4 mg/kg at 0, 12 and 24 hours, then daily thereafter. Formulate a plan which may involve delivery with senior members of the multi-disciplinary team, including consultant physician and obstetrician.

F   Admit to hospital, administer oral chloroquine 600 mg followed by 300 mg 68 hours later, followed by 300 mg on day 2 and day 3, administer anti-emetics and make a plan with the multi-disciplinary team for management of recurrence and future antenatal care/delivery.

OBSTETRICS

11

G   Postpone any treatment until after delivery, which
    should be planned for the same day, administer steroids
    and liaise with the neonatal team.
H   Terminate pregnancy.

**Match the most appropriate management
to the scenario:**

16  A 27-year-old woman who is 32 weeks pregnant
    presents following a recent trip abroad with vomiting
    and flu-like symptoms, but with no pyrexia. She has
    been seen by the Acute Medical team and diagnosed
    with malaria (*p. falciparum*).
17  A 30-year-old woman who is 28 weeks pregnant
    presents following a recent trip abroad with vomiting
    and flu-like symptoms, but with no pyrexia. She has
    been diagnosed with *p. vivax* malaria by the Acute
    Medical team.
18  A 27-year-old woman is 26 weeks pregnant and
    presents with vomiting and pyrexia. She is found to be
    hypoglycaemic and to have severe anaemia. Blood
    pressure is 80/50 mmHg and pulse rate 120.
    *P. falciparum* is found on testing.

# PREVENTION AND MANAGEMENT OF POSTPARTUM HAEMORRHAGE

## Options

A  Misoprostol 1000 mcg rectally
B  Oral ampicillin and metronidazole
C  Oral clindamycin
D  Surgical evacuation of uterus/retained products
E  IV oxytocin 5 IU
F  IM oxytocin 5 or 10 IU
G  Carboprost 0.25 mg IM
H  Pelvic ultrasound
I  Surgical evacuation of uterus/retained products with consultant supervision and IV antibiotics
J  Conservative management of the third stage (physiological third stage)
K  IM oxytocin and ergometrine
L  MRI scan

**Match the most appropriate management to each scenario:**

19  A 27-year-old woman in her first pregnancy with no identifiable risk factors for PPH delivers vaginally. What should be offered for management of the third stage of labour?

20  A 32-year-old woman presents with mild vaginal bleeding 10 days post normal delivery. She is well in herself with no pyrexia. She has no allergies. What is the most appropriate next step?

21  A 34-year-old woman presents with heavy vaginal bleeding five days post normal delivery. The woman is pyrexial and has been commenced on oral antibiotics by the GP, however is not responding to treatment. On admission, her blood pressure is 90/50 mmHg and her pulse rate is 120. On examination, she has a tender uterus. What is the most appropriate next step?

OBSTETRICS

## MANAGEMENT OF SICKLE CELL DISEASE IN PREGNANCY

### Options

A  Penicillin
B  Influenza vaccine
C  Refer to haematologist
D  Folic acid 5 mg
E  Hydroxycarbamide (hydroxyurea)
F  Iron
G  Prophylactic antibiotics
H  Pertussis vaccine
I  Undertake a further test to assess iron levels
J  Angiotensin converting enzyme inhibitors (ACE inhibitors)
K  Non-steroidal anti-inflammatory drugs (NSAIDs)
L  Hydroxycarbamide (hydroxyurea) and continue contraception for three months

### Match the most appropriate drug or advice to the scenario outlined:

22  A 33-year-old woman with sickle cell disease presents to the pre-conception clinic. She would like to become pregnant and her partner has already been tested for sickle cell disease (which is negative). The woman is taking a number of medications and is advised to stop a particular drug at least three months prior to conception.

23  A 28-year-old woman with sickle cell disease is 16 weeks pregnant. She attends the antenatal clinic and is seen jointly by the haematologist and the obstetrician. She has been taking folic acid since the beginning of her pregnancy. She is advised to attend her general practitioner to obtain a substance that is a prophylactic measure that she has not had in the last 12 months.

24  A 29-year-old woman with sickle cell disease is 14 weeks pregnant. She is seen by the midwife in antenatal clinic to discuss the results of her blood tests from her booking appointment. She is Rubella immune, negative for syphilis and HIV, and her haemoglobin is 8.4 g/dL.

# SUTURING MATERIALS

## Options

A   Polydiaxanone (PDS) 3–0
B   Polyester (Dacron)
C   Polyglactin (Vicryl Rapide)
D   Polyglycolic acid (Dexon)
E   Polypropylene (Prolene)
F   Polyglyconate (Maxon)
G   Polyamide (Nylon)
H   Polydiaxanone (PDS) 2–0

## Match the most appropriate suture type to each scenario:

25   A suture material used to repair an episiotomy.
26   A suture material used to repair the internal or external anal sphincter.

# RASH AND INFECTIOUS DISEASE IN PREGNANCY

## Options

A   Test for measles IgG
B   Test for measles IgM and IgG
C   Test for parvovirus IgG
D   Test for parvovirus IgM and IgG
E   Test for varicella zoster virus (VSV) IgG
F   Test for rubella IgG
G   Test for rubella IgM and IgG
H   Test for varicella zoster virus (VZV) IgM
I   Reassure and wait for a rash to appear

## Match the appropriate initial management plan to each scenario:

27   A 25-year-old woman is 22 weeks pregnant and her 2-year-old daughter has had a chickenpox rash for the past three days. As far as she can remember, the woman has not had chickenpox as a child.

28   A 30-year-old schoolteacher is 18 weeks pregnant and several children have reported to her that they have developed a rash. On further examination by the school nurse, the rash is not thought to be chickenpox. The teacher is concerned by the undiagnosed rash, but knows that she is immune to measles and rubella from childhood vaccinations.

OBSTETRICS

17

# PLACENTA PRAEVIA AND ACCRETA

## Options

A Transvaginal ultrasound scan
B MRI scan
C Refer to a unit with cell salvage and/or interventional radiology
D Crossmatch four units of blood
E Admit for observation
F Consent for hysterectomy
G Autologous blood transfusion
H Elective caesarean section at 38 weeks of gestation
I Discuss with haematologist and blood bank

## Match the most appropriate management plan to each scenario:

29 A 32-year-old, para 1 Jehovah's Witness is 34 weeks pregnant. She has had one previous caesarean section. Ultrasound scan shows an anterior placenta, 1.5 cm from the internal os with an irregular retroplacental sonolucent zone and abnormal placental lacunae. Colour Doppler shows hypervascularity between the bladder and serosa interface.

30 A 33-year-old woman para 0 is 37 weeks pregnant. She is known to have a placenta praevia. She has had minimal bleeding in her pregnancy and on abdominal palpation, the fetal head is now engaged.

# AIR TRAVEL AND PREGNANCY

## Options

A  No additional risk
B  Low-dose aspirin
C  Graduated elastic compression stockings
D  Low-molecular-weight heparin for the day of travel
E  Low-molecular-weight heparin for the day of travel and several days after
F  High-dose low-molecular-weight heparin
G  Avoid flight after 32 weeks of gestation
H  Avoid flight after 37 weeks of gestation
I  Avoid flight after 34 weeks of gestation
J  Avoid flight altogether

## Match the most appropriate advice to each scenario:

31  A 27-year-old woman presents to the antenatal clinic when she is 28 weeks pregnant. She is concerned about her risk of venous thromboembolism during her forthcoming six hour flight to the USA. She has no additional risk factors or known thrombophilia.

32  A 28-year-old woman is 26 weeks pregnant in her first pregnancy, carrying monochorionic diamniotic twins. She wishes to fly to Australia.

33  A 32-year-old woman is 28 weeks pregnant and wishes to fly to the USA. Her booking haemoglobin was 9.0 g/dl and she has been on iron; however, at 28 weeks, her haemoglobin is 7.0 g/dl.

# MANAGEMENT OF SMALL FOR GESTATIONAL AGE FETUSES

## Options

A   Uterine artery Doppler at 20–24 weeks
B   Assessment of fetal size and umbilical artery Doppler at 26–28 weeks, followed by serial ultrasound assessment
C   Assessment of fetal size and umbilical artery Doppler in third trimester
D   Deliver by caesarean section
E   Biophysical profile
F   Administer corticosteroids and deliver
G   Cardiotocograph (CTG)
H   Ductus venosus Doppler
I   Induction of labour
J   Middle cerebral artery (MCA) Doppler

## Match the most appropriate management to each scenario:

34   A 36-year-old woman presents to antenatal clinic in her first pregnancy, with a body mass index (BMI) of 27. She has no medical problems but doesn't have a particularly balanced diet with minimal fruit and vegetable intake. Uterine artery Doppler at 20 weeks is normal.

35   A 25-year-old woman is referred to antenatal clinic in her first pregnancy at 30 weeks of gestation by the midwife who measured her symphysis fundal height and found this to be small for her gestational age. An ultrasound scan indicated that the fetus was growing on the ninth centile. Umbilical artery Doppler at 29 weeks is normal. Fetal movements are reported as normal by the mother. Umbilical artery Doppler is repeated two weeks later and the Doppler is found to be absent. Ductus venosus Doppler is performed and found to be absent.

# UMBILICAL CORD PROLAPSE

## Options

A  Deliver immediately by caesarean section (category 1)
B  Artificial rupture of membranes
C  Admit to hospital
D  Artificial rupture of membranes in theatre/controlled setting
E  Speculum/digital vaginal examination
F  Deliver by caesarean section (category 2)
G  Operative vaginal birth
H  Breech extraction
I  Knee–chest position
J  Left lateral position

## For each scenario, what would be your initial management/advice?

36  You are the on-call doctor for obstetrics. A community midwife calls to alert you to the fact that she has a patient delivering at home with an umbilical cord prolapse. She tells you that she is in established labour, her cervix is 5 cm dilated and she is multiparous. She is currently travelling via ambulance with the patient to the hospital.

37  A multiparous woman (para 2) is in spontaneous labour with a singleton pregnancy. The emergency buzzer is pressed by the midwife to alert the team to the fact that there has been a cord prolapse. On examination, you find that there is no head palpable abdominally, the cervix is fully dilated and the fetal head is 1 cm below the ischial spines, no caput with a small amount of moulding.

38  A primiparous woman is in spontaneous labour with a singleton pregnancy. Labour has been progressing well and on vaginal examination one hour ago by the midwife, the patient's cervix was 5 cm dilated.

You are called into the labour room by the midwife as the cardiotocograph is now showing fetal heart rate variable decelerations, following artificial rupture of membranes.

39  A primiparous woman at 32 weeks of gestation is admitted to hospital following spontaneous rupture of membranes. Clear liquor is draining, but the woman is not experiencing any contractions. She is administered a corticosteroid injection.
A cardiotocograph is commenced and shows fetal heart rate variable decelerations.

# GYNAECOLOGY

# MANAGEMENT OF GENITO-URINARY PROLAPSE

## Options

A   Anti-cholinergics
B   Treatment of prolapse
C   Botulinum toxin to bladder
D   Defer surgery until bladder stable
E   Discussion at multi-discliplinary team meeting
F   Referral to tertiary urogynaecology centre
G   Counselling regarding after-effects of surgery
H   Surgery first and then treat overactive bladder symptoms
    later on
I   Do nothing
J   Treat urodyamnic stress incontinence and detrusor
    overactivity simultaneously
K   Referral to urologist

**Match the most appropriate management
to each scenario:**

40   A 51-year-old woman presents with mainly irritative
     symptoms and occasional stress incontinence and her
     reason for referral is bothersome prolapse. These are the
     results of her urodynamic studies: flow rate 50 ml/min,
     urgency at 162 ml, strong urgency at 308 ml, no
     urodynamic stress incontinence, definite sensory
     urgency and phasic detrusor contractions after standing
     up with full bladder.

41   A 57-year-old woman presents with a cystocele (no
     vault descent) and urgency symptoms. Urodynamics
     were performed with pessary *in situ* at 50 ml/min,
     filled to 500 ml; urodynamic stress incontinence not
     demonstrated due to sustained pressure rise, but definite
     detrusor overactivity observed.

42   A 52-year-old woman presents with mixed symptoms;
     urodynamics performed on detrusitol, at 50 ml/min,

bladder could not be filled beyond 376 ml, strong urge and urgency at 328 ml, poor compliance and severe urodynamic stress incontinence, blood-stained post void residual.

43  A 43-year-old woman, who had a total abdominal hysterectomy three years ago and lower urinary tract symptoms ever since, underwent urodynamic investigation. The study at 50 ml/min shows stable bladder during filling phase and severe urodynamic stress incontinence, but an after-contraction just after voiding.

44  A 74-year-old woman with a previous history of vaginal hysterectomy and anterior repair presents with severe irritative symptoms (mostly urgency) on maximum anticholinergics. Urodynamic studies at 50 ml/min show severe detrusor overactivity with no urodynamic stress incontinence.

# MANAGEMENT OF EARLY PREGNANCY PROBLEMS

## Options

A   Complete miscarriage
B   Delayed miscarriage
C   Ectopic pregnancy
D   Pregnancy of unknown location
E   Persistent pregnancy of unknown location
F   Pregnancy of uncertain viability
G   Threatened miscarriage
H   Ruptured ectopic
I   Missed miscarriage
J   Viable pregnancy
K   Threatened miscarriage

## Match the most appropriate diagnosis to each scenario:

45   A 27-year-old woman presents to the early pregnancy assessment unit via her GP with very irregular periods and uncertain last menstrual period (LMP), but maybe about seven weeks ago. Transvaginal scan reveals a sac with mean sac diameter (MSD) of 19 mm, but no fetal pole and no yolk sac. There is no adnexal abnormality, but minimal fluid in the pouch of Douglas (POD).

46   A 33-year-old woman with a BMI of 43 presents to the early pregnancy unit with mild bleeding and a positive pregnancy test. Serum human chorionic gonadotrophin (hCG) is 1100 IU, which rises to 1800 and then to 3300; each of these were done 48 hours apart. Transvaginal ultrasound scans reveals thickened endometrium with fluid in POD. Diagnostic laparoscopy could not identify any ectopic pregnancy in the tubes.

47   A 43-year-old woman presented to the early pregnancy unit with amenorrhoea of 7–8 weeks and having passed

something at home with pain and bleeding, which seems to be settling. Speculum examination reveals a slightly open os. Scan confirms a thickened endometrium and hCG of 3900 IU. Neither adnexae could be identified properly due to gas in bowel; however, there was echogenic free fluid in the POD.

48  A 22-year-old woman was seen in the early pregnancy unit with amenorrhoea, minimal bleeding and some pain. hCG was 1350 IU. Scan revealed a sac in the uterus containing an embryo with crown–rump length (CRL) 8.6 mm, but no fetal heart noticed.

49  A 32-year-old woman complains of upper abdominal pain and bleeding at 9 weeks of gestation by date, although her periods are quite irregular. She has a previous history of right-sided ectopic pregnancy. HCG done by GP was 1300 IU, approximately 36 hours ago. Repeated hCG of 1600 IU and transvaginal scan suggested multiple fibroids in uterus, the largest one in the right cornu, about 6 cm in diameter with thickened endometrium. hCG repeated 48 hours later was 3000 IU, but still no sign of an intrauterine sac.

50  A 26-year-old woman, para 1 (previous caesarean section), presents with a history of abdominal pain and minimal bleeding. hCG was measured at 3270 IU. Transvaginal scan suggested a complex mass on the right ovary 51 × 42 × 67 mm, which looked more like an endometriotic cyst, although not definitive, and echogenicity in the POD.

# POSTOPERATIVE COMPLICATIONS

## Options

A    CT urogram
B    IVP
C    Ultrasound scan
D    CT scan of abdomen and pelvis
E    Full blood count
F    V/Q scan
G    Urea and electrolytes
H    Cystogram
I    Venous leg Doppler
J    Chest X-ray
K    Abdominal X-ray
L    Urinary catheterisation
M    Intermittent self catheterisation

## Match the most appropriate management to each scenario:

51    A 48-year-old woman had a total abdominal hysterectomy and bilateral salpingo-oophorectomy for a suspicious-looking ovarian cyst. There was significant ascites of 1.5 litres. Postoperative recovery was uneventful; however, she was re-admitted with lower abdominal pain and leakage of fluid per vaginum.

52    A 67-year-old woman had a hysteroscopy and drainage of pyometra. Twelve hours postoperatively, the woman was significantly pyrexial and very unwell.

53    Twelve hours after having a TVT procedure, a patient complains of inability to pass urine after the removal of an indwelling urinary catheter.

54    A 26-year-old woman had a perforation of her bladder during a trans-vaginal tape (TVT) operation.

55    Seven days after a total abdominal hysterectomy and bilateral salpingo-oophorectomy for grade

1 endometrial cancer, a 72-year-woman was admitted with swinging pyrexia and renal angle tenderness.

56 A 42-year-old woman had a total abdominal hysterectomy and left salpingo-oophorectomy three weeks ago. Admitted with severe left-sided abdominal pain, an ultrasound scan of her pelvis was inconclusive, but the possibility of left-sided hydronephrosis was raised, which was thought to be moderate.

# CHRONIC PELVIC PAIN

## Options

A  Non-steroidal anti-inflammatory
B  Danazol
C  Oral contraceptive pills
D  LUNA
E  Mebeverine hydrochloride
F  Diagnostic laparoscopy
G  Referral to urologist
H  Screen for sexually transmitted infection
I  Referral for counselling
J  Gastroenterology referral
K  Referral to pain team
L  Gabapentin

GYNAECOLOGY

## Match the most appropriate management to each scenario:

57  A 34-year-old woman with irregular vaginal bleeding and postcoital bleeding complains of chronic pelvic pain.

58  A 38-year-old woman complains of heavy menstrual bleeding. An ultrasound scan was highly suggestive of an endometrioma on the left adnexa.

59  A 23-year-old woman has recently been complaining of lower abdominal pain. She says she is in a new relationship and is finding it hard to have penetrative sex. You notice that during the whole consultation she is not maintaining eye contact at all.

60  A 64-year-old woman complains of lower abdominal pain and pain when typically the bladder fills up. Ultrasound scan suggested a small cyst on the left ovary.

61  A 58-year-old woman had a trans-obturator vaginal tape procedure (TOT) about 12 months ago. She has been complaining of groin pain on the left side for some time now, which started about six weeks after the

procedure. The pain radiates down the back of thigh and she feels as if there is an electric current that passes down the leg.

62  A 26-year-old woman referred by her GP complains of lower abdominal pain for over 12 months. She has also been complaining of recent onset bleeding per rectum and feels that the pain occasionally gets better with the passage of stools.

# FERTILITY PROBLEMS

## Options

A   Ovarian stimulation with clomiphene citrate
B   Referral to specialist fertility centre
C   In-vitro fertilisation (IVF)
D   Intrauterine insemination (IUI)
E   IUI with ovarian stimulation
F   Single embryo transfer
G   Double embryo transfer
H   Triple embryo transfer
I   Gamete intra-fallopian transfer (GIFT)
J   Zygote intra-fallopian transfer (ZIFT)
K   Cryopreservation

**From the options above, name the fertility treatment or option that you would NOT use:**

63   A couple has been trying for a pregnancy for over 24 months now. She has normal periods and tests have confirmed ovulation and her tubes are patent. Her partner's semen analysis has been found to be normal as well. They live a healthy lifestyle and are obviously worried about the next step.

64   A couple has been trying for a baby for 13 months now. Tests have shown the woman is ovulating and her partner's semen analysis has come back as normal. Due to the pain associated with her periods, a diagnostic laparoscopy and dye test showed bilateral tubal spillage, but there was evidence of mild endometriosis.

65   A 36-year-old lady is having her second full cycle of IVF and was wondering how many embryos will be transferred.

66   A 41-year-old lady with unexplained infertility is having her first full cycle of IVF and wants to know how many embryos will be transferred.

67 A 38-year-old with unexplained infertility is having her third cycle of IVF and wishes to maximize her chances of pregnancy.

68 A 35-year-old woman with normal periods has had tests for ovulation and tubal patency and both have come back as normal. Her partner's semen analysis has shown mild problems with the total sperm count on two occasions.

# NON-PHARMACOLOGICAL TREATMENT OF MENOPAUSAL SYMPTOMS

## Options

A   Vitamin E
B   Soy
C   Red clover
D   Black cohosh
E   Evening primrose oil
F   Ginseng
G   Ginko biloba
H   Phytoestrogen

**Match the most appropriate treatment to each scenario:**

69   A 48-year-old woman has been reading about a plant-based phytoestrogen that has been shown in placebo-controlled studies to be superior to placebo in controlling vasomotor symptoms and would like to use it instead of hormone replacement therapy (HRT).

70   A 54-year-old woman has used HRT for five years now and would like to change over to a non-pharmacological product. She has selected a product that seems to contain a legume-based phytoestrogen which hasn't shown a statistically significant benefit over placebo in meta-analysis.

71   A 49-year-old woman with previous treatment for breast cancer would like to use a compound, but has been searching for information on the internet and has found that it can act as selective estrogen receptor modulator and may cause potential harm in estrogen-dependent tumours and antagonise the response of tamoxifen.

72   A 56-year-old woman has been using a product for a few years now with good effect; however, she has

heard that this compound can cause problems with
platelet aggregation.

73  A 53-year-old woman has heard about a product and is
anxious that this might only give a modest benefit of
reducing only one flush per day.

# PRECOCIOUS PUBERTY

## Options

A   Thyroxine
B   Glucocorticoids
C   Glucocorticoids with mineralocorticoids
D   Hydrocortisone
E   Testosterone
F   Anastrozole
G   GnRH analogue therapy
H   Medroxyprogesterone acetate
I    Tamoxifen
J   Ketoconazole
K   Spironolactone
L   Cyproterone acetate
M   Multi-disciplinary team meeting (MDT)

**GYNAECOLOGY**

## Match the most appropriate management to each scenario:

74   An 11-year-old girl has been referred by her GP, having started her periods more than 18 months ago. On examination, she has hyperpigmented macules in certain parts of her body with features of axillary and pubic hair as well as breast enlargement. Her GP has referred her for a bone scan, which she has already had, but hasn't been made aware of the results.

75   A young couple has been referred as their newborn baby boy doesn't seem to be gaining weight and in fact, when weighed by the health visitor seems to have had more than 10% weight loss. The baby is quite dehydrated on examination and has just vomited. The couple is also worried about the size of the baby's penis.

76   A 14-year-old girl has been referred with primary amenorrhoea. She seems to have a deep voice with a lot of acne and has also been harassed in school because of excessive hair on her body.

77 A 12-year-old girl has presented to A and E with significant abdominal pain and vaginal bleeding. Examination reveals a mass arising from the pelvis, which is confirmed on scan, showing a cyst containing suspicious and solid elements. The girl admits to previous similar bleeding that she has never told her mother about and says she is sexually inactive.

78 A three-month-old child is seen with normal birth weight and length. The mother states that the baby is often drowsy, has a hoarse-sounding cry, difficulties with feeding and constipation. You also notice an enlarged tongue, umbilical hernia, dry skin, a decreased body temperature and jaundice.

# VULVAL LESIONS

## Options

A  Behcet's syndrome
B  Lichen planus
C  Apthous ulcer
D  Candidiasis
E  Lichen sclerosus
F  Vulval intraepithelial neoplasia (VIN)
G  Vaginal intraepithelial neoplasia (VAIN)
H  Anal intraepithelial neoplasia (AIN)
I  Syphilitic ulcer
J  Herpetic lesion
K  Lichenoid skin reaction

## Match the most appropriate diagnosis to each scenario:

79  A 36-year-old woman presents with vulval lesions in the form of small red papules, which are flat topped and shiny with white streaks on top.

80  A 54-year-old woman presents with irregular pigmented plaques causing a burning sensation and significant itching around the vulva.

81  A 20-year-old woman presents with significant vaginal discharge, not foul-smelling, occasionally causing itching, with some fissuring and superficial ulceration, but mostly erythematous.

# MEDICAL MANAGEMENT OF URINARY INCONTINENCE

## Options

A   Intermediate release (IR) oxybutynin
B   Mirabegron
C   Darifenacin
D   Oxybutynin patches
E   Solifenacin
F   Topical oestrogen
G   Desmopressin
H   Imipramine
I   Duloxetine
J   Fesoterodine
K   Tamsulosin
L   Botulinum toxin
M   Discussion at multi-disciplinary team meeting
N   Percutaneous tibial nerve stimulation (PTNS)

## Match the most appropriate management to each scenario:

82  A 64-year-old woman was referred with irritative symptoms of mostly urgency symptoms. Fluid advice was given, as she was drinking about six cups of coffee a day, which mostly corrected the problem. Pelvic examination revealed severe atrophic vaginitis.

83  A 59-year-old woman presents with significant and bothersome urgency and urge incontinence and passes urine six times during the day. However, nocturia was her most bothersome symptom. A trial of anti-muscarinic medication controlled her daytime frequency and urgency, but her nocturia has persisted.

84  A 36-year-old woman is bothered by urgency and urge incontinence. Fluid advice and bladder retraining have been advocated and she has already had a trial of three anti-cholinergic medications. Although she had some

improvement with the medication, the tablets were not able to control all of her symptoms and she has had to discontinue her medication due to side-effects.

85   A 23-year-old woman has had a long-standing problem with nocturnal enuresis. She has tried an alarm system and desmopressin in the past with limited success. She would like to try something else, if available.

86   A 42-year-old woman has tried both solifenacin and tolterodine and although both have been successful in controlling her symptoms, she is having very bad side-effects, with both dry mouth and constipation, and would like something else to control her symptoms.

# USE OF ANTIBIOTICS

## Options

A   Cephalosporin
B   Cephalosporin + metronidazole
C   Doxycycline
D   Flucloxacillin
E   Amoxacillin with clavulanic acid
F   Vancomycin
G   Ofloxacin + metronidazole + doxycycline
H   Discuss with microbiologist
I   Ticarcillin
J   Meropenem
K   Metronidazole

## Match the most appropriate management to each scenario:

87   An 18-year-old woman presents with a vulval swelling, which she thinks has grown slightly bigger and is painful. She is apyrexial and not unwell.

88   A 20-year-old woman has been admitted through the gynaecology assessment unit with lower abdominal pain and discharge. Examination revealed very tender adnexae and raised inflammatory markers.

89   A 56-year-old woman had a vaginal hysterectomy and anterior repair 48 hours ago and is complaining of lower abdominal pain, feeling unwell and borderline pyrexia.

90   A 48-year-old woman had an endometrial ablation carried out 24 hours ago and has been re-admitted with swinging pyrexia.

91   A 41-year-old woman had a total abdominal hysterectomy and bilateral salpingo-oophorectomy for suspected adenomyosis of uterus. She was pyrexial immediately after the procedure and was prescribed cephalosporin intravenously. Her pyrexia failed to settle after 24 hours of intravenous therapy.

# INDICATIONS FOR EMERGENCY CONTRACEPTION

## Options

A  Take both missed pills, take the remaining pills as usual, condoms should be used for the next seven days or sexual intercourse avoided in case further pills are missed. No indication for emergency contraception.

B  Take the most recent missed pill, take the remaining pills as usual, condoms should be used for the next seven days or sexual intercourse avoided in case further pills are missed. No indication for emergency contraception.

C  Administer the next injection, offer emergency contraception, additional contraception or abstinence should be advised for the next seven days and a pregnancy test should be carried out in 21 days.

D  Take both missed pills, take the remaining pills as usual, condoms should be used for the next seven days or sexual intercourse avoided in case further pills are missed. Emergency contraception should also be advised.

E  The next injection should not be administered, emergency contraception should be offered and a pregnancy test should be carried out in 21 days.

F  Administer the next injection, emergency contraception not required, additional contraception or abstinence for the next seven days.

## Match the most appropriate advice to each scenario:

92  A 28-year-old woman misses two consecutive 30 mcg combined pills in the second week of taking her packet (days 9 and 10). She has been taking all her pills on days 1–7. She had sexual intercourse with her boyfriend on day 8.

93   A 32-year-old woman had her last DMPA
     (Depo-Provera) injection 14 weeks and two days
     ago. She had sexual intercourse with her partner two
     days ago.

# HEAVY MENSTRUAL BLEEDING

## Options

A    Levonorgestrel intrauterine system
B    Uterine artery embolisation
C    Internal iliac artery embolisation
D    Hysteroscopic resection
E    Myomectomy
F    Abdominal hysterectomy
G    Vaginal hysterectomy
H    GnRH analogues for three months prior to
     hysterectomy
I    Endometrial ablation

## Match the most appropriate treatment to each scenario:

94    A 28-year-old woman has multiple fibroids (all greater
      than 3 cm in diameter), which are causing pressure pain
      and heavy menstrual bleeding. She has been trying
      to conceive for the past three years. She understands
      and accepts surgery for complications.

95    A 27-year-old woman wishes to have a procedure
      that has the best evidence for future fertility following
      treatment for fibroids.

96    A 45-year-old woman has had period problems
      throughout her life. She has multiple fibroids, the
      largest of which is 4 cm in diameter. She has had two
      normal vaginal deliveries in the past.

# CONTRACEPTION PROBLEMS

## Options

A   Leave in for a further 12 months and then remove or check two FSH (follicular stimulating hormone) levels, six weeks apart, and if both over 30 IU/L, remove.

B   Take a full sexual history and commence a 30 mcg or 35 mcg combined oral contraceptive pill. If not resolving, consider endometrial biopsy.

C   Take a full sexual history and investigate for sexually transmitted infections if appropriate.

D   Take a full sexual history and a cervical smear.

E   Stop the contraceptive and advise trying a long-acting reversible contraceptive such as the implant.

F   Take a full sexual history, do a pelvic examination and cervical smear. If normal, consider adding mefenamic acid alongside.

G   Remove the device now.

H   Leave in for a further 24 months and then remove or check two FSH levels six weeks apart and if both over 30 IU/L, remove after 12 months.

**Match the most appropriate management to each scenario:**

97   A 43-year-old woman started a combined oral contraceptive pill three months ago. She has started having irregular bleeding. She is known to have PCOS (polycystic ovarian syndrome). She is a non-smoker and is up to date with her smears.

98   A 24-year-old woman presents with irregular bleeding six months after starting the combined oral contraceptive pill. She has no medical problems. She has recently started a new relationship. She is up to date with her smears.

99   A 50 year old woman has used the levonorgestrel IUS (intrauterine system) for heavy menstrual bleeding for

the past five years and is amenorrhoeic. She now wonders whether she has gone through the menopause, and therefore can have the coil removed.

100  A 52-year-old woman had a copper coil fitted at the age of 43. Her last menstrual period was 13 months ago. She wishes to know whether she has gone through the menopause and therefore can have the coil removed.

# COLPOSCOPY AND CERVICAL SMEARS

## Options

A  Repeat smear in six months
B  Colposcopy in the second trimester to exclude high-grade pathology
C  Wedge biopsy
D  Repeat smear in three years
E  Repeat smear 3–4 months postnatally
F  Refer for urgent colposcopy
G  Cone biopsy
H  Large loop excision of the transformation zone (LLETZ)
I  Repeat smear in 12 months
J  Refer for colposcopy

## Match the most appropriate management plan to each scenario:

101  A 27-year-old woman is 24 weeks pregnant in her first pregnancy. She had been on routine three-yearly smears prior to her pregnancy when one had been found to show mild dyskaryosis, two months before she found herself to be pregnant.

102  A 39-year-old woman, para 0, is a renal dialysis patient. She has a routine smear and the result indicates evidence of mild dyskaryosis.

103  A 35-year-old woman is diagnosed with HIV. Her routine smear result comes back as normal. A colposcopy also indicates no evidence of cervical pathology.

# MANAGEMENT OF CERVICAL CARCINOMA

## Options

A  Radiotherapy
B  Repeat smear in six months
C  LLETZ (large loop excision of the transformation zone)
D  Radiotherapy and chemotherapy
E  Postmenopausal bleeding pathway
F  Trachelectomy
G  Radical surgery with radiotherapy
H  No further treatment
I  See and treat LLETZ
J  Repeat LLETZ
K  LLETZ with follow-up
L  Follow-up smears
M  Cone biopsy
N  NETZ (needle excision of the transformation zone)

## Match the most appropriate management to each scenario:

104  A 26-year-old nulliparous woman has been trying to conceive for 12 months. Her routine smear showed the presence of possible cancer cells. Colposcopy and biopsy reveals a lesion limited to the cervix, measuring 3.9 cm.

105  A 38-year-old woman was referred by her GP with a smear result showing severe dyskaryosis. Colposcopic biopsy revealed the presence of CIN III (cervical intraepthelial neoplasia). A LLETZ was performed and histopathology revealed a cervical cancer with a depth of 3 mm and horizontal spread of 6 mm, with clear margins.

106  A 32-year-old nulliparous woman was very anxious, as her recent smear suggested severe dyskaryosis. Further colposcopy confirmed high-grade disease.

GYNAECOLOGY

107 A 63-year-old woman was referred with very heavy bleeding per vaginum. She has never had a smear in her life and on examination, a large mass was noticed around the cervix with bleeding emanating from this mass. Vaginal packing wasn't able to control the bleeding.

108 A 38-year-old nulliparous woman has been trying for a pregnancy for well over a year now. Her recent smear has suggested the presence of cancer cells. Colposcopy and biopsy reveals a lesion $4.7 \times 5.9$ cm in size. She is very keen on having a family.

# RECURRENT MISCARRIAGE

## Options

A   Low-dose aspirin
B   Referral to geneticist
C   Progesterone supplementation
D   Cervical cerclage
E   Human chorionic gonadotrophin (hCG) supplementation
F   Low-dose aspirin and low-molecular-weight heparin
G   Immunoglobulin therapy
H   Uterine septum resection
I    Metformin
J   Emotional/psychological support

## Match the most appropriate management to each scenario:

109  A couple are referred to the recurrent miscarriage clinic following their third recurrent miscarriage before 10 weeks of gestation. The woman is aged 39 and the man is aged 42. The couple have no history of medical problems. Cytogenetic analysis from their last miscarriage indicated an unbalanced chromosomal arrangement. Parental karyotype has been taken and the father has been found to carry a balanced Robertsonian translocation.

110  A couple are referred to the recurrent miscarriage clinic following their third recurrent miscarriage before 10 weeks of gestation. The woman is aged 36 and the man is aged 45. The couple have no history of medical problems. Screening has indicated the presence of anti-phospholipid antibodies in the woman. She has no history of thromboembolism.

111  A couple are referred to the recurrent miscarriage clinic following their third recurrent miscarriage before

GYNAECOLOGY

10 weeks of gestation. The woman is aged 27 and the man is aged 32. The couple have no history of medical problems. Cytogenetic analysis has revealed no genetic abnormality. Serum screening has revealed no abnormality. Pelvic ultrasound is normal.

# OUTPATIENT HYSTEROSCOPY: BEST PRACTICE

## Options

A   Use opiate-based analgesia
B   Use a non-steroidal anti-inflammatory drug one hour before the procedure
C   Offer a chaperone
D   Use normal saline as the distension medium
E   A chaperone is not needed as the doctor is female
F   The choice of distension medium is at the discretion of the operator
G   Use carbon dioxide as the distension medium
H   Apply local anaesthetic topically to the ectocervix

## Match the most appropriate guidance to each scenario:

112   A 43-year-old woman is attending the outpatient hysteroscopy service for investigation of intermenstrual bleeding. She has no medical problems. She is concerned about the level of discomfort following the procedure.

113   A 62-year-old woman is attending the outpatient hysteroscopy service for investigation of postmenopausal bleeding. She has no medical problems. Dr Green (a female doctor) is the doctor undertaking the procedure and the woman feels at ease with the doctor following her explanation of the procedure.

114   A 45-year-old woman is the attending the outpatient hysteroscopy service for the removal of an endometrial polyp which has been seen on ultrasound scan. She has no medical problems or allergies. The doctor performing the procedure decides to perform electrosurgery (cautery) to remove the polyp.

# HYSTEROSCOPY AND ENDOMETRIAL PATHOLOGY

## Options

A  Perform annual screening for endometrial cancer
B  Perform hysteroscopy +/− polypectomy
C  Offer levonorgestrel intrauterine system
D  Consider changing contraception, if any, then wait and see
E  Reassure
F  Offer vaginoscopic-approach outpatient hysteroscopy
G  Offer hysteroscopy under general anaesthetic
H  Offer hysterectomy
I  None of the above

## Match the most appropriate management to each scenario:

115  A 66-year-old woman who has never had penetrative sex has been referred to your clinic with a history of vaginal spotting, visible on wiping. She has an anxiety disorder. Ultrasound scan of her pelvis reveals endometrial thickening to 15 mm and cystic spaces within it. There is also fluid distension of the uterine cavity.

116  A 76-year-old woman with a history of receptor negative breast cancer has recurrent endometrial polyps on scan. She has had these removed twice and is now fed up. Medically, she is not ideally suited for major surgery in view of previous multiple thromboembolic events.

117  A 38-year-old para 1 is seen in your clinic with intermenstrual bleeding. Apart from a proliferative pattern endometrium, there is nothing remarkable on hysteroscopy or histology. She reveals to you that she has been seen at the genetics clinic owing to her family history and diagnosed to have HNPCC (hereditary

non-polyposis colorectal cancer syndrome). She is keen to keep her childbearing options open.

118 A 90-year-old woman is referred with vaginal spotting. Her ultrasound suggests fluid separation of the endometrium by 1.2 mm and cumulative 3.8 mm. Her ovaries are not visualised clearly. In clinic, she is noted to have dementia and is heavily dependent on carers.

119 A 40-year-old woman complains of recurrent intermenstrual and postcoital bleeding. She has had an outpatient hysteroscopy on two occasions in the last two years and these have been reported as entirely normal. She reports having been on Depo-Provera for the last four years.

GYNAECOLOGY

# MANAGEMENT OF VULVAL SKIN DISORDERS

## Options

A   Skin patch testing
B   Clobetasol
C   Immunomodulators
D   Topical anti-fungal cream
E   $CO_2$ laser vaporisation
F   Local excision
G   Simple vulvectomy
H   Radical vulvectomy
I   General measures
J   Laser therapy
K   HPV vaccination
L   Immunosuppressants
M   Interferon therapy
N   Photodynamic therapy

## Match the most appropriate management to each scenario:

120   A 53-year-old woman presents with severe pruritus and thinning of the vulval skin, which bleeds on scratching. There is pain, discomfort and dyspareunia and adhesion of the labial margins on examination. She also suffers from diabetes.

121   A 33-year-old woman presents with recent onset of irritation and soreness of the vulva but with a long-standing history of vaginal discharge. There is also evidence of an inflamed area on the inner side of the thigh.

122   A 42-year-old woman presents with recurrent oral and genital ulcers, which are quite painful. There is extensive evidence of scarring from previous lesions.

123   Significant pruritus in a 52-year-old smoker with red plaques and some warty lesions.

124  A 32-year-old woman presents with vulval lesions that are smooth and discrete, red in colour, but not affecting the vaginal mucosa. The patient also complains of discrete lesions in the flexural areas of the body.

125  A 44-year-old woman complains of a long-standing history of inflammatory bowel disease and complains of recent onset swelling and ulceration of the vulva and occasionally something draining out of these swollen areas.

# MISCELLANEOUS

# TEACHING METHODS

## Options

A   The Delphi technique
B   The one-minute preceptor
C   Problem-based learning
D   Schema activation
E   Complex procedural hierarchy
F   Schema refinement
G   Snowballing
H   Lectures
I   Peer coaching

## Which teaching method is being described in each scenario?

126   A group of medical students learn together as a group using a theoretical case of a gynaecology patient. They read through the case, discuss potential themes and create learning objectives incorporating physiological, psychological, anatomical, ethical and professional aspects, amongst other themes. The role of the tutor is as a facilitator to ensure that the students do not discuss themes at a tangent to the case.

127   A group of obstetrics and gynaecology trainees attend a tutorial by their consultant on the physiology and endocrinology of polycystic ovarian syndrome. The tutor then provides real-life examples of cases of women affected by the condition and the group discusses how to solve their clinical problems.

128   An obstetric trainee begins to learn how to perform a caesarean section by assisting his consultant. The consultant and trainee develop a rapport over a period of time, leading to the consultant assisting the trainee to perform their first caesarean section. Eventually, through ongoing assessment and feedback, the trainee

performs the caesarean section with another trainee assisting, supervised by the consultant.

129 A group of obstetrics and gynaecology trainees ask their consultant for a tutorial about current fertility treatments. The tutor wishes to know the trainees' current knowledge and understanding of the subject so that she can further their knowledge with her tutorial and therefore, asks the trainees questions first to build a discussion that subsequently influences what she includes in her tutorial.

# CAPACITY AND THE MENTAL HEALTH ACT

## Options

A   Advance directive
B   Living will
C   Advance refusal
D   Advance decision
E   Lasting power of attorney
F   Court of protection
G   Mental Capacity Act (2005)
H   Consult relevant persons to determine the best interests of the patient

**With each scenario, what is the most relevant part of the Mental Health Act?**

130   A 32-year-old woman is a Jehovah's Witness. She has a placenta praevia at 36 weeks of gestation and is to have a planned caesarean section for delivery of the baby. She refuses all blood products; this has been discussed with her in antenatal clinic and a form has been signed so that all relevant healthcare professionals understand her wishes.

131   An 82-year-old woman is diagnosed with stage 4 endometrial cancer. Treatment is palliative. She pre-emptively decides to appoint her son to make decisions with regard to her medical treatment if her health deteriorates to a point where she lacks capacity to make decisions herself.

132   A 72-year-old woman has stage 3 ovarian cancer and treatment is palliative. She has been admitted to the medical ward following a stroke, but the medical team are now ready to discharge the patient. The medical team have asked you to review the patient to make a plan of care following discharge; however, the patient is unable to communicate with you with regard to her wishes for the rest of her care.

# PROVIDING INFORMATION ABOUT RISK

## Options

A  Very common (1/1–1/10)
B  Common (1/10–1/100)
C  Frequent (1/25–1/50)
D  Uncommon (1/100–1/1000)
E  Rare (1/1000–1/10 000)
F  Very rare (Less than 1/10 000)
G  Never event

## Match the most appropriate risk group to each scenario:

133  A 43-year-old woman has been advised by the consultant to undergo a total abdominal hysterectomy for menorrhagia, after all other treatment options have failed. She has a BMI of 23 and has never had any previous abdominal surgery and has no medical problems. She wishes to know what her risk is of damage to bladder or ureter.

134  A 23-year-old woman with a BMI of 22 is to undergo a planned caesarean section for breech presentation of her baby. She has had no previous abdominal surgery. She wishes to know what her risk is of damage to her bladder or ureter.

135  A 38-year-old woman has a screening test for Down's syndrome and based upon the result, is offered an amniocentesis. The risks of the procedure are discussed with her and she wishes to know what her risk of sepsis (chorioamnionitis) is.

# DECISION-MAKING AT SURGERY

## Options

A   Ask a specialist colleague to take a look at the mass at the time of surgery, before removing the mass
B   Remove the mass at the time of surgery
C   Leave the mass alone, abandon the procedure and discuss with the patient once she is awake, including referral for a specialist opinion
D   Leave the mass alone, abandon the procedure and discuss with the patient once she is awake, then re-list for your next available theatre slot
E   Perform an oophorectomy
F   Perform a salpingectomy
G   Perform a tubal ligation (sterilisation)

## Match the most appropriate management to each scenario:

136   A 48-year-old woman is undergoing total abdominal hysterectomy and bilateral salpingo-oophorectomy for pelvic pain and premenstrual syndrome. She has a BMI of 33, no previous abdominal surgery but is a known diabetic (Type I). Unexpectedly, a large mass is found which appears to be arising from the right ovary.

137   A 23-year-old woman is undergoing a diagnostic laparoscopy for chronic pelvic pain. She has a BMI of 28, had one previous caesarean section and is known to have irritable bowel syndrome. She is using a copper coil for contraception. Unexpectedly, a mass is seen that appears to be within the left tube, which has a blue-ish tinge and appears to be rupturing through the tube.

## ASSESSMENT AND FEEDBACK

### Options

A  Formative assessment
B  Appraisal
C  Summative assessment
D  Evaluation
E  Construct validity
F  Face validity
G  Content validity
H  Feedback
I  Predictive criterion validity

### Match the most appropriate descriptor to each scenario:

138  An ST5 trainee is preparing her e-portfolio for her end of year meeting with her tutors. She has to ensure that she has included all her assessments that she has completed over the past 12 months to show that she has achieved the standards expected of her for the year of training. She receives feedback on her performance to date and new goals for the coming year are established.

139  An ST2 trainee meets with his educational supervisor following undertaking his first caesarean section, whilst being assisted by a junior colleague. His educational supervisor was observing his performance. His supervisor provides helpful comments about his performance, focussing on the positives, but also providing constructive criticism so that he may learn how to improve his performance.

140  An ST6 trainee is undertaking the Advanced Training Specialty Module (ATSM) in medical education. He provides a small group of medical students with tutorials every week based upon topics in obstetrics and gynaecology. At the end of the semester, he asks them to provide written feedback about the tutorials and his teaching performance.

# STATISTICS

## Options

A   0.23
B   0.50
C   1.95
D   1.66
E   0.60
F   0.95
G   0.62
H   1.12
I   0.05
J   1.62
K   5.00
L   1.05
M   0.03

A cohort study is carried out to ascertain the association between smoking and cervical cancer. The total number of women recruited is 1000; 500 are smokers and 500 non-smokers. The table below gives the results at follow-up after 20 years:

|  | Cervical cancer | No cervical cancer | Total |
|---|---|---|---|
| Smokers | 34 | 466 | 500 |
| Non-smokers | 21 | 479 | 500 |
| Total | 55 | 945 | 1000 |

141   What is the relative risk of cervical cancer in smokers? (correct to two decimal places)
142   This result is reported to be significant at the 5% level. What is the correct $p$ value?

# STATISTICS

## Options

A  Positive predictive value
B  Test positive
C  Incidence density
D  Sensitivity
E  True negative
F  Negative predictive value
G  Attributable risk
H  Incidence
I  Relative risk
J  Period prevalence
K  Cumulative incidence
L  Specificity
M  Point prevalence

An antenatal screening test was carried out on 1000 pregnant women, 42 of whom tested positive. It was later found that 18 of these pregnancies were actually affected with the condition, with a total of 21 affected pregnancies in the original group.

143  A doctor, after reading the study, tells his patient, "The condition affects about two percent of pregnancies." What is the figure he is quoting?
144  A researcher does the following calculation: 956/979 = 97.7% What does this figure represent?
145  The researcher then does the following calculation: 956/959 = 99.7% What does this figure represent?

# SURGERY IMPROVING FERTILITY OUTCOMES AND UNDERSTANDING STATISTICS

## Options

A   Twofold increase in success rate
B   3.5-fold increase in success rate
C   Odds ratio of 1.6
D   Conception rate of 35–84%
E   Spontaneous conception rate of 50%
F   Odds ratio of 2.06
G   Fivefold increase in conception rate
H   <40 mm
I   >40 mm
J   <60 mm
K   >60 mm
L   No difference in conception rate at 12 and 24 months
M   Odds ratio of 4

## Match the most appropriate answer to each scenario:

146  A Cochrane review of three RCTs suggested treatment with GnRH analogue for a period of 3–6 months prior to IVF for endometriosis leads to increased odds of clinical pregnancy.

147  The Endometriosis Canadian Multi-centre (ENDOCAN) RCT showed an increase in conception rate following laparoscopy and treatment of superficial endometriosis compared to diagnostic laparoscopy alone.

148  Conception rate following hysteroscopic adhesiolysis of intrauterine adhesions.

149  Laparoscopic salpingectomy for treatment of hydrosalpinx identifiable and clearly visible on ultrasound scan showed an increase in conception rate.

150  Office hysteroscopy just prior to IVF treatment increases clinical pregnancy rate.

# ANSWERS

# RHESUS D PROPHYLAXIS

*Source*: RCOG Green Top Guideline No 22: The use of anti-D immunoglobulin for Rhesus D prophylaxis (April 2011)

1 **Answer**: B – Kleihauer and 500 IU anti-D

*Explanation*: Anti-D IgG is given to all non-sensitised Rhesus negative women who experience a potentially sensitising event (i.e. where maternal and fetal blood may potentially mix). This prevents maternal allo-immunisation, which may not necessarily affect the first pregnancy, but more likely, subsequent pregnancies. At or after 20+0 weeks, a minimum dose of 500 IU anti-D should be administered to the woman as an intramuscular injection. 500 IU is enough to protect up to 4 ml of potential feto-maternal haemorrhage. A Kleihauer test should be used at this stage to identify a greater amount than this and therefore advise upon further doses of anti-D.

2 **Answer**: F – Anti-D at six-weekly intervals

*Explanation*: Recurrent bleeding is a difficult situation in which to appropriately counsel a mother; however, RCOG guidance advises repeat anti-D at six-weekly intervals for recurrent bleeding.

3 **Answer**: J – Check antibody screen at booking and at 28 weeks

*Explanation*: Maternal allo-immunisation can still occur, even when there has been no recognised sensitising event. This is thought to be due to a 'silent' feto-maternal haemorrhage. Routine antenatal anti-D prophylaxis (RAADP) was introduced to try to combat such effects and there is evidence that RAADP does reduce such incidence, hence its introduction into antenatal care.

However, some women will decline RAADP (e.g. those who wish to be sterilised after birth) and women should be counselled with regard to risks and benefits so that an informed decision can be made. In such cases, the antibody screen should be checked at booking and 28 weeks to look for any sensitising events.

4  **Answer**: G – Large dose (2500 IU or 5000 IU) anti-D required

*Explanation*: If less than 15 ml has been transfused, the appropriate dose of anti-D (based on a Kleihauer test) should be administered. If more than 15 ml has been transfused, it is likely that a large dose will need to be given.

# CHICKENPOX IN PREGNANCY

*Source*: RCOG Green Top Guideline No 13: Chickenpox in pregnancy (September 2007)

5   **Answer**: F – Administer VZIG and manage as potentially infectious from 8–28 days after administration

*Explanation*: Of the population in the UK and Ireland, 90% are immune to chickenpox (primary varicella zoster virus infection) as it is a common childhood disease. Immunity is not routinely tested for antenatally, nor is immunisation routine. It can cause fetal varicella syndrome in pregnancy (albeit rare), but can also cause maternal morbidity and mortality in non-immune individuals.

If an individual is known to be non-immune (sero-negative), a history should be undertaken to determine significant exposure, defined as in the same room for at least 15 minutes, face-to-face contact and contact in a large open ward.

VZIG should then be given as soon as possible, but within 10 days of the contact – this may prevent or attenuate the disease in pregnant women (this immunoglobulin is derived from non-UK donors with high VSV antibody titres). Women should then be treated as potentially infectious for 8–28 days after administration (8–21 days if no VZIG given).

6   **Answer**: C – No risk

*Explanation*: Maternal shingles occurs as a secondary infection in an individual who has previously had chickenpox. As the woman has already acquired antibodies to VSV and these will transfer across the placenta to the baby *in utero*, there is no risk to the neonate at birth and no treatment or monitoring is required. The exceptions are if the baby is born before

28 weeks (as antibodies will not have transferred across the placenta) or if the baby weighs less than 1 kg.

7 **Answer**: H – Administer VZIG and monitor for 28 days after administration

*Explanation*: If maternal disease occurs seven days before or after delivery, there is a risk of varicella in the newborn; therefore, the neonate should be given VZIG, again to try to attenuate the disease. Although 50% of neonates still develop chickenpox, mortality appears to be lower. VZIG can prolong the incubation period and therefore neonates should be monitored for signs of infection for 28 days and acyclovir administered as necessary.

# REDUCING THE RISK
# OF THROMBOEMBOLISM

*Source:* RCOG Green Top Guideline No 37a: Thrombosis and embolism during pregnancy and the puerperium, reducing the risk (November 2009)

8  **Answer**: C – Antenatal high-dose LMWH and six weeks postnatal LMWH

*Explanation*: Getting the appropriate type and dose of LMWH can be very tricky to remember, and in a clinic setting, memory should not be relied upon and information always clarified with a local or national guideline such as the RCOG. There is a handy table in Appendix 2 of the RCOG guideline which would be useful to remember for the exam.

Individuals with anti-thrombin deficiency are at very high risk of thromboembolism (therefore high-dose LMWH is usually necessary), but different types of anti-thrombin deficiency are associated with different levels of risk, therefore, an expert haematologist should also be involved with the care of the woman.

Read the options carefully as it is easy to miss the words 'high-dose'!

9  **Answer**: B – Antenatal LMWH and six weeks postnatal LMWH

*Explanation*: Some studies have shown that a previous oestrogen (from pregnancy or the oral contraceptive pill)-provoked venous thromboembolism is a risk factor for recurrence, whilst others have not. RCOG guidance advises, however, that these women should be offered antenatal and postnatal LMWH.

Generally, women with a previous VTE from any cause do have a risk of recurrence, both during pregnancy and in the postpartum period. An antenatal risk assessment should always be undertaken to identify any additional risk factors.

10   **Answer**: H – Seven days postnatal LMWH

*Explanation*: Both obesity (BMI > 30) and smoking are risk factors for venous thromboembolism. The RCOG guideline has an excellent flow chart to help stratify individual risk factors to determine whether LMWH is required or not. In this case, as two risk factors are present, if admitted the patient would require antenatal LMWH – however, generally seven days postnatal LMWH only would be required (thromboembolism risk increases in the postnatal period due to relative increase in coagulation factors).

# THE ACUTE MANAGEMENT OF THROMBOSIS AND EMBOLISM

*Source*: RCOG Green Top Guideline No 37b: The acute management of thrombosis and embolism in pregnancy and the puerperium (February 2007, reviewed 2010)

11 **Answer**: G – Bilateral lower limb Doppler

*Explanation*: Venous thromboembolism has been an important cause of death of pregnant women in many of the recent maternal mortality reports.

Investigations in this situation are all about balancing risk to the fetus and to the mother. Chest X-rays are of negligible risk to the fetus, but may show other causes of shortness of breath. If the chest X-ray is negative, the next step would be to perform a bilateral lower limb Doppler as the presence of a deep vein thrombosis (DVT) would make the diagnosis of pulmonary embolism highly likely. CTPA and V-Q scan are both associated with risks to mother and/or fetus.

Treatment-dose, low-molecular-weight heparin should be commenced prior to the results of these investigations, unless there is a contra-indication.

12 **Answer**: H – Anti-Xa level

*Explanation*: Therapeutic doses of low-molecular-weight heparin are given to women based on their pre-pregnancy or booking weight. Satisfaction with treatment is based on anti-Xa levels and most women achieve good therapeutic coverage if guidelines are adhered to.

However, factors such as extremes of body weight (over 90 kg or less than 50 kg), recurrent thrombo-embolism or renal impairment may alter effectiveness, and monitoring of anti-Xa is advised.

# HYPERTENSION IN PREGNANCY

*Source*: NICE Clinical Guideline 107: Hypertension in pregnancy (August 2010, modified January 2011)

There is a useful table within the guideline that can be used to answer these questions.

13  **Answer**: A – Do not admit patient to hospital or treat hypertension; no indication for blood tests, but monitor blood pressure weekly.

*Explanation*: Treating hypertension in pregnancy and trying to deduce the risks of pre-eclampsia can be very challenging. NICE guidance in 2010 went some way to try to stratify risk and guide clinicians as to when to admit/treat etc.

By definition in the NICE guidance, this patient has mild gestational hypertension (and not pre-eclampsia) – i.e. they have raised blood pressure without significant proteinuria. The patient is at risk of developing pre-eclampsia in the future, but does not need treatment nor admission at this stage – however, blood pressure should be monitored weekly.

14  **Answer**: E – Admit patient to hospital, treat hypertension with oral anti-hypertensives, take blood pressure at least four times per day and take a quantificative protein test.

*Explanation*: By NICE definition, this patient has moderate pre-eclampsia and therefore needs admission, treatment and further investigations.

Once a quantificative protein test has been taken, it does not need to be repeated and it is merely the presence of protein that is being assessed and not an increase.

Oral labetalol would be first-line management in the treatment of hypertension, aiming to keep the systolic less than 150 mmHg and the diastolic between 80 and 100 mmHg.

15 **Answer**: F – Admit patient to hospital, treat hypertension with alternate including IV anti-hypertensives, take blood pressure at least four times per day and take a quantificative protein test. Consider the administration of steroids, discuss with consultant obstetrician, neonatal and anaesthetic staff with regards to delivery.

*Explanation*: The patient was managed according to NICE guidance in the first instance; however, the patient's blood pressure has become refractory to treatment and she may need early delivery if it is not able to be controlled – balancing the risk to the fetus against the benefits of continuing with the pregnancy.

# THE DIAGNOSIS AND TREATMENT OF MALARIA IN PREGNANCY

*Source*: RCOG Green Top Guideline 54b: The diagnosis and treatment of malaria in pregnancy (April 2010)

16 **Answer**: B – Admit to hospital, administer oral quinine 600 mg 8-hourly and oral clindamycin 450 mg 8-hourly for seven days, administer anti-emetics and make a plan with the multi-disciplinary team for management of recurrence and future antenatal care/delivery.

*Explanation*: It is advisable to hospitalise all pregnant women with malaria (especially *P. falciparum*), as women can deteriorate rapidly. Women should be managed jointly by the medical and obstetric teams – delay in diagnosis and treatment can be fatal.

If vomiting is persistent, oral therapy should be changed to IV. Women should also be screened for anaemia and treated.

Primaquine should not be used in pregnancy.

17 **Answer**: F – Admit to hospital, administer oral chloroquine 600 mg followed by 300 mg 68 hours later, followed by 300 mg on day 2 and day 3, administer anti-emetics and make a plan with the multi-disciplinary team for management of recurrence and future antenatal care/delivery.

*Explanation*: Management is as in the first scenario; however, this is a different species causing malaria and therefore, requires a different agent.

18 **Answer**: E – Admit to Intensive Care Unit and administer artesunate IV 2.4 mg/kg at 0, 12 and 24 hrs, then daily thereafter. Formulate a plan which may

involve delivery with senior members of the multi-disciplinary team, including consultant physician and obstetrician.

*Explanation*: This woman has severe malaria with complications and requires urgent admission to the Intensive Care Unit. Hypotension may also indicate secondary bacterial infection. Once again, a multi-disciplinary approach should be taken, which may involve delivery of the baby.

# PREVENTION AND MANAGEMENT OF POSTPARTUM HAEMORRHAGE

*Source*: RCOG Green Top Guideline No 52: Prevention and management of postpartum haemorrhage (May 2009, with minor revisions in November 2009 and April 2011)

19 **Answer**: F – IM oxytocin 5 or 10 IU

*Explanation*: This may seem like an easy question and answer, however many obstetric units in the UK actually use a mixture of oxytocin and ergometrine, as it does reduce the risk of minor postpartum haemorrhage (PPH), but it increases the risk of vomiting. Oxytocin alone is the first-line choice, as it has similar efficacy at this level of PPH without the adverse side-effects of the combined drug.

Conservative management could be offered, however the guideline states that all women should be offered prophylactic oxytocics to reduce PPH.

20 **Answer**: B – Oral ampicillin and metronidazole

*Explanation*: The most common cause of secondary postpartum haemorrhage is infection or endometritis, which is easily treated with oral antibiotics. The unit in which you are working will probably have local guidelines, however RCOG recommend the ones above.

Pelvic ultrasound would not change the management of this situation (see below).

21 **Answer**: I – Surgical evacuation of uterus/retained products with consultant supervision and IV antibiotics

*Explanation*: This woman presents with overt sepsis and it is likely that retained products are the cause. She needs a surgical evacuation, however there is a high risk of perforation when the procedure is completed shortly after birth – therefore, senior supervision is required. Intravenous antibiotics will be required and RCOG recommends the use of gentamicin in this situation.

Pelvic ultrasound would not alter management and is an unreliable tool in scenarios of secondary postpartum haemorrhage due to the appearance of the postpartum uterus, where retained products can be difficult to distinguish from the uterus and endometrium itself.

# MANAGEMENT OF SICKLE CELL DISEASE IN PREGNANCY

*Source*: RCOG Green Top Guideline No 61: Management of sickle cell disease in pregnancy (July 2011)

22 **Answer**: L – Hydroxycarbamide (hydroxyurea) and continue contraception for three months

*Explanation*: Hydroxycarbamide is used to reduce sickle cell crises; however, it is teratogenic and women should be advised to stop the drugs at least three months prior to conception. Contraception should also therefore be continued at the same time. Remember to read all the way down the list of options!

ACE inhibitors should also be stopped prior to conception; however, there is no specific guidance that this needs to be at least three months before.

23 **Answer**: B – Influenza vaccine

*Explanation*: Women with sickle cell disease are hyposplenic and therefore, much more prone to infection. Penicillin prophylaxis is used throughout pregnancy and women should have an annual influenza vaccine (as should all pregnant women).

24 **Answer**: I – Undertake a further test to assess iron levels

*Explanation*: Anaemia may not necessarily be due to iron deficiency in women with sickle cell disease – in fact the woman may be iron overloaded due to repeated blood transfusions. In this situation, iron supplementation would be the wrong advice to give. A further test to assess iron levels is the right answer here before iron supplementation, if appropriate.

# SUTURING MATERIALS

*Source*: RCOG Green Top Guideline No 29: The management of third degree and fourth degree perineal tears (March 2007)

25  **Answer**: C – Polyglactin (Vicryl Rapide)

*Explanation*: A fast-absorbing braided suture is used for second degree perineal tears and episiotomies

26  **Answer**: A – Polydiaxanone (PDS) 3–0

*Explanation*: A fine suture should be used for the internal or external anal sphincter to reduce irritation and discomfort. From the list, monofilament PDS 3–0 is the most appropriate and named within the guideline.

# RASH AND INFECTIOUS DISEASE IN PREGNANCY

*Source*: Guidance on viral rash in pregnancy: Investigation, diagnosis and management of viral rash illness, or exposure to viral rash illness, in pregnancy. Health Protection Agency (January 2011)

With these questions, the answers are not as simple as they seem. You have to be clear on what you are testing for and why.

27 **Answer**: E – Test for varicella zoster virus (VZV) IgG

*Explanation*: Many women born in the UK are immune to chickenpox as they were exposed to the illness in childhood. However, it is important to ascertain immunity if the woman is unsure.

The presence of IgG indicates past infection and the woman can be reassured.

28 **Answer**: D – Test for parvovirus IgM and IgG

*Explanation*: Parvovirus needs to be excluded here. It is a relatively easily transmissible disease and outbreaks occur commonly in nurseries or schools.

As asymptomatic parvovirus can affect the unborn child just as much as symptomatic parvovirus, and active management of the disease can alter the outcome for the child, it is important to test the woman for current infection and for immunity.

The presence of IgM usually indicates current infection, with IgG showing past infection. Further testing is sometimes advised if the initial test shows neither the presence of IgM nor IgG.

# PLACENTA PRAEVIA AND ACCRETA

*Source*: RCOG Green Top Guideline No 27: Placenta praevia, placenta praevia accreta and vasa praevia: diagnosis and management (January 2011)

29 **Answer**: C – Refer to a unit with cell salvage and/or interventional radiology

*Explanation*: With a previous caesarean section and ultrasound features typical of placenta accreta, this woman is at high risk of postpartum haemorrhage. As she is a Jehovah's witness and most likely refuses blood transfusion, which would be confirmed with a discussion with the patient and the completion of an advance directive, the woman should be referred to a unit with cell salvage and/or interventional radiology so that a planned elective caesarean section can be performed at around 38 weeks with these extra modalities to reduce blood loss at surgery.

30 **Answer**: A – Transvaginal ultrasound scan

*Explanation*: Whilst many women deliver by caesarean section with a placenta praevia, the evidence for this is thin and more research is required. Therefore, if the head is engaged, there is a place for transvaginal ultrasound scan to see if vaginal delivery may be an option. Decisions regarding mode of delivery should always encompass clinical factors as well as the woman's preferences.

# AIR TRAVEL AND PREGNANCY

*Source*: RCOG Scientific Impact Paper 1: Air Travel and Pregnancy (May 2013)

31 **Answer**: C – Graduated elastic compression stockings

*Explanation*: Whilst there is a small absolute risk of venous thromboembolism during a flight, combined with the risks of pregnancy, this risk is increased for pregnant women, especially in flights over four hours.

General advice, including good fluid intake and mobilisation, reduce the risk and all women undertaking a flight over four hours should wear compression stockings.

32 **Answer**: G – Avoid flight after 32 weeks of gestation

*Explanation*: The main risk with air travel in pregnancy is the risk of labour and facilities not being available to provide care for women in labour, or the risk of the plane being diverted.

Therefore, women with additional risk factors for pre-term labour such as multiple pregnancy are generally advised not to travel after 32 weeks.

33 **Answer**: J – Avoid flight altogether

*Explanation*: There are certain conditions, such as sickle cell disease or recent gastrointestinal surgery or haemoglobin below 7.5 g/dl that can lead to an increased risk of complications with air travel during pregnancy.

The patient should be advised not to travel in these circumstances.

# MANAGEMENT OF SMALL FOR GESTATIONAL AGE FETUSES

*Source*: RCOG Green Top Guideline No 31: The management of the small for gestational age fetus (second edition, Feb 2013)

34 **Answer**: C – Assessment of fetal size and umbilical artery Doppler in third trimester

*Explanation*: These relatively new guidelines from the RCOG recommend that women should have an assessment of risk factors for a small for gestational age (SGA) fetus at booking. Four minor risk factors (here: low fruit intake, age above 35, first pregnancy and BMI 25–29) recommend a uterine artery Doppler at 20 weeks followed by a third trimester ultrasound assessment if the uterine artery Doppler is normal.

35 **Answer**: F – Administer corticosteroids and deliver

*Explanation*: Whilst umbilical artery Doppler has minimal benefit in a low-risk population, it is an important tool in a case where an SGA fetus has been identified. Umbilical artery Doppler measures the resistance to blood flow between baby and placenta. Where this remains normal, Doppler can be assessed every 14 days.

Ductus venosus Doppler can then be used as an adjunct, if umbilical artery Doppler then becomes abnormal, and can be used to plan delivery. Ductus venosus Doppler reflects atrial pressure–volume changes during the cardiac cycle.

Gestational age is critical to survival and the administration of corticosteroids for lung maturity is also critical to this survival.

ANSWERS

# UMBILICAL CORD PROLAPSE

*Source*: RCOG Green Top Guideline No 50: Umbilical cord prolapse (April 2008)

36 **Answer**: J – Left lateral position

*Explanation*: Knee–chest position is often adopted when a woman is at home, to relieve pressure of the presenting part on the cord. However, in a moving ambulance, this position is thought to be more dangerous and therefore, left lateral should be adopted.

There are, of course, other measures that can be used by the midwife to relieve pressure of the presenting part, such as manual elevation or filling the urinary bladder.

37 **Answer**: G – Operative vaginal birth

*Explanation*: Whilst an immediate caesarean section (Grade 1) is often the way many babies are delivered following a cord prolapse, if it is deemed safe and quicker to do so, an operative vaginal birth may be carried out. However, it should be borne in mind that if the delivery is not successful, delay will then be compounded by having to then carry out a caesarean section.

38 **Answer**: E – Speculum/digital vaginal examination

*Explanation*: A change in fetal heart rate monitoring following artificial rupture of membranes is characteristic of an umbilical cord prolapse. A vaginal examination should be carried out to confirm this and make plans for delivery.

39  **Answer**: E – Speculum/digital vaginal examination

*Explanation*: Whilst with pre-term rupture of membranes it is often best to avoid examination and therefore infection, in this scenario, an umbilical cord prolapse may have occurred and examination will influence the management plan and delivery.

# MANAGEMENT OF GENITO-URINARY PROLAPSE

*Source*: NICE Clinical Guideline 171: Urinary incontinence in women (September 2013)

40 **Answer**: D – Defer surgery until bladder stable

*Explanation*: Whilst prolapse has been the reason for referral, urodynamics have uncovered bladder problems, which need to be stabilised prior to surgery and not made worse.

41 **Answer**: A – Anti-cholinergics

*Explanation*: Once again, her bladder symptoms need to be stabilised, this time with anti-cholinergics.

42 **Answer**: E – Discussion at multi-disciplinary team meeting

*Explanation*: In this situation, mixed urinary incontinence has been revealed. Blood-staining post residual may highlight something sinister or more complex, and therefore a multi-disciplinary team meeting is warranted.

43 **Answer**: G – Counselling regarding after-effects of surgery

*Explanation*: After-contractions of the bladder observed during voiding cystometry may worsen following surgery and be indicative of *de novo* detrusor overactivity – therefore, this needs to be discussed prior to surgery.

44 **Answer**: E – Discussion at multi-disciplinary team
     meeting

*Explanation*: There is evidence here of detrusor overactivity
on maximum dosage of anti-cholinergics. The next step may
be administration of botulinum toxin; however, NICE
guidance suggests multi-disciplinary team discussion before
this decision is made.

# MANAGEMENT OF EARLY PREGNANCY PROBLEMS

*Source*: NICE Clinical Guideline 154: Ectopic pregnancy and miscarriage (December 2012)

45  **Answer**: F – Pregnancy of uncertain viability

*Explanation*: MSD <25 mm with a trans-vaginal scan with no visible fetal pole and/or yolk sac signifies a pregnancy of uncertain viability and a second scan needs to be performed after seven days before making a diagnosis.

46  **Answer**: E – Persistent pregnancy of unknown location

*Explanation*: Although there are increasing levels of hCG, signifying a pregnancy in an unknown location, there is a negative laparoscopy making the diagnosis difficult. This is a case of persistent PUL, which is a difficult one to treat as there is always a niggling doubt about a viable pregnancy and, hence, instituting methotrexate treatment becomes difficult. Good communication with the patient is key to successful management.

47  **Answer**: C – Ectopic pregnancy

*Explanation*: Presence of echogenic fluid on an ultrasound scan should always raise the possibility of blood/clots in the pouch of Douglas. This along with an empty uterus and a significantly raised hCG level should always alert us to the possibility of an ectopic pregnancy.

48  **Answer**: I – Missed miscarriage

*Explanation*: CRL >7 mm with a transvaginal ultrasound scan without a visible heartbeat signifies a missed miscarriage.

However a second opinion should be sought and a second scan can be offered after seven days before making a diagnosis.

49 **Answer**: D – Pregnancy of unknown location

*Explanation*: In this case there is a risk factor of previous ectopic pregnancy, hence we should be very careful in our diagnosis. A conservative approach should be applied and appropriate counselling should be offered. The presence of fibroids makes early pregnancy scanning difficult. Although there is a high index of suspicion of an ectopic, pregnancy of unknown location is the diagnosis until proven otherwise.

50 **Answer**: C – Ectopic pregnancy

*Explanation*: Again, echogenicity in the pouch of Douglas makes the diagnosis easy, along with a complex mass in the adnexa. This situation warrants a diagnostic laparoscopy for the patient.

**ANSWERS**

# POSTOPERATIVE COMPLICATIONS

These questions aim to assess your ability to detect postoperative complications and how to manage them. The difficulty with this is that different hospitals and departments may manage these complications in different ways – therefore do not be too disheartened if you feel that more than one answer could be true!

There isn't a particular guideline to quote, but experience gathered from best practice. This particular section is aimed at giving candidates from outside the UK a flavour of how to deal with postoperative complications.

51  **Answer**: A – CT urogram

*Explanation*: A vesicovaginal or ureterovaginal fistula needs to be ruled out as a complication by the use of this investigation.

52  **Answer**: D – CT scan of abdomen and pelvis

*Explanation*: Uterine perforation may have occurred.

53  **Answer**: M – Intermittent self catheterisation

*Explanation*: Minor postoperative voiding difficulty is not uncommon and contrary to resting the bladder with an indwelling catheter, it is better to get the bladder to work by performing ISC.

54  **Answer**: L – Urinary catheterisation

*Explanation*: Resting the bladder with an indwelling catheter is appropriate. If a major perforation is suspected, performing a cystogram is justified.

55 **Answer**: D – CT scan of abdomen and pelvis

*Explanation*: This investigation would be used to look for bowel perforation.

56 **Answer**: B – IVP

*Explanation*: This investigation would be used to look for ureteric injury.

# CHRONIC PELVIC PAIN

*Source*: RCOG Green Top Guideline No 41: The initial management of chronic pelvic pain (May 2012)

57 **Answer**: H – Screen for sexually transmitted infection

*Explanation*: Chronic pelvic pain is frequently encountered in clinical practice. Postcoital bleeding together with chronic pelvic pain can be a sign of a sexually transmitted infection and therefore, genito-urinary swabs should be taken.

58 **Answer**: F – Diagnostic laparoscopy

*Explanation*: This patient may be managed conservatively, however, the fact that she has sought medical attention for her heavy periods and the fact that there is no mention of the size of the endometrioma, a diagnostic laparoscopy could be offered.

59 **Answer**: I – Referral for counselling

*Explanation*: This question is trying to make you think about domestic or sexual abuse and therefore, an empathetic approach would be appropriate with consented referral for counselling.

60 **Answer**: G – Referral to urologist

*Explanation*: This is interstitial cystitis and therefore, referral to the urologist is appropriate.

61 **Answer**: K – Referral to pain team

*Explanation*: This scenario is suggestive of postoperative nerve injury. Whilst gabapentin may be an option, this is best prescribed with the support and guidance of the specialist pain team.

62 **Answer**: J – Gastroenterology referral

*Explanation*: This is most likely irritable bowel syndrome and mebeverine could be commenced. However, in light of the associated bleeding, a referral to the gastroenterologist should be made.

# FERTILITY PROBLEMS

*Source*: NICE Clinical Guideline 156: Fertility (February 2013)

63  **Answer**: A – Ovarian stimulation with clomiphene citrate

*Explanation*: Do not offer oral ovarian stimulation agents to women with unexplained infertility – there are risks of ovarian hyperstimulation and multiple pregnancy, and these may not be of benefit in women with unexplained infertility (Section 1.8.1.1 of the guideline).

64  **Answer**: C – In-vitro fertilisation

*Explanation*: IVF should be offered following two years of trying to conceive naturally (1.9.1.1).

65  **Answer**: G – Double embryo transfer

*Explanation*: Single embryo transfer is preferred to minimise the risks of multiple pregnancy. Double embryo transfer may be considered if embryos are of poor quality or in a number of special circumstances (see below).

66  **Answer**: F – Single embryo transfer

*Explanation*: At age 40–42, double embryo transfer may be considered (1.12.6.5).

67  **Answer**: F – Single embryo transfer

*Explanation*: At age 37–39, single embryo is advocated in the first and second cycles, but in the third, it is suggested to use no more than two embryos.

68 **Answer**: D – Intrauterine insemination

*Explanation*: The couple should be advised to try to conceive for at least two years before any referral for fertility treatment should be made. IUI should not be used without concurrent ovarian stimulation (1.9.1.1).

# NON-PHARMACOLOGICAL TREATMENT OF MENOPAUSAL SYMPTOMS

*Source:* Tong I. Non-pharmacological treatment of postmenopausal symptoms. *The Obstetrician and Gynaecologist* 2013; **15**: 19–25.

69 **Answer**: B – Soy

*Explanation*: Soy is a plant-based phyto-oestrogen and used by many women to try to control menopausal symptoms, especially vasomotor symptoms.

70 **Answer**: C – Red clover

*Explanation*: There is no evidence that red clover is significantly better than placebo.

71 **Answer**: B – Soy

*Explanation*: Soy can interestingly counteract tamoxifen as it is a phyto-oestrogen.

72 **Answer**: C – Red clover

*Explanation*: Red clover can cause problems with platelet aggregation.

73 **Answer**: A – Vitamin E

*Explanation*: Vitamin E has been shown only to have moderate benefit in reducing vasomotor symptoms.

# PRECOCIOUS PUBERTY

*Source:* Tirumuru S.S. *et al.* Understanding precocious puberty in girls. *The Obstetrician and Gynaecologist* 2012; **14**: 121–129.

74   **Answer**: F – Anastrozole

*Explanation*: This is McCune–Albright syndrome and is treated with an aromatase inhibitor.

75   **Answer**: C – Glucocorticoids with mineralocorticoids

*Explanation*: This is classical congenital adrenal hyperplasia.

76   **Answer**: D – Hydrocortisone

*Explanation*: This is a non-classical form of congenital adrenal hyperplasia, treated with hydrocortisone.

77   **Answer**: M – MDT meeting

*Explanation*: This may be an oestrogen-secreting tumour such as a granulosa cell tumour.

78   **Answer**: A – Thyroxine

*Explanation*: The baby appears to have congenital primary hypothyroidism.

# VULVAL LESIONS

Vulval lesions and their characteristics and treatment are often the subject of both EMQs and MCQs.

79 **Answer**: B – Lichen planus

80 **Answer**: J – Herpetic lesion

81 **Answer**: A – Behcet's syndrome

# MEDICAL MANAGEMENT OF URINARY INCONTINENCE

*Source*: NICE Clinical Guideline 171: Urinary incontinence in women (September 2013)

82 **Answer**: F – Topical oestrogen

*Explanation*: As this woman is postmenopausal and has atrophic vaginitis, topical oestrogen may help improve all her symptoms.

83 **Answer**: G – Desmopressin

*Explanation*: Isolated nocturia is rare and difficult to treat. Desmopression should only be used after a detailed consultation and estimation of serum urea and electrolytes.

84 **Answer**: M – Discussion at multi-disciplinary team meeting

*Explanation*: Botulinum toxin may be the next step, but discussion at an MDT meeting should occur, as suggested by the guideline.

85 **Answer**: H – Imipramine

*Explanation*: Nocturnal enuresis is difficult to treat and requires a stepwise approach – there is further NICE guidance on nocturnal enuresis.

86 **Answer**: D – Oxybutynin patches

*Explanation*: Patches are a good option to avoid side-effects such as dry mouth etc.

ANSWERS

## USE OF ANTIBIOTICS

Anti-microbial protocols vary in hospitals, so it is worth getting to know the system in your own hospital.

87  **Answer**: D – Flucloxacillin

*Explanation*: This is a Bartholin's abscess.

88  **Answer**: G – Ofloxacin + metronidazole + doxycyline

*Explanation*: This is pelvic inflammatory disease.

89  **Answer**: B – Cephalosporin + metronidazole

*Explanation*: This is a common postoperative complication and ideally a broad spectrum antibiotic should be used.

90  **Answer**: B – Cephalosporin + metronidazole

*Explanation*: This is a common postoperative complication and ideally a broad spectrum antibiotic should be used.

91  **Answer**: H – Discuss with microbiologist

*Explanation*: A multi-disciplinary team approach must be applied, as this patient is unresponsive to initial treatment.

# INDICATIONS FOR EMERGENCY CONTRACEPTION

*Source*: Faculty of Sexual and Reproductive Healthcare Clinical Effectiveness Unit statements: Missed pill recommendations (May 2011) and Progestogen-only injectable contraception (June 2009)

92 **Answer**: B – Take the most recent missed pill, take the remaining pills as usual, condoms should be used for the next seven days or sexual intercourse avoided in case further pills are missed. No indication for emergency contraception.

*Explanation*: Missed pill guidance can be very complex to remember and it's important that you remember every detail to ensure that you choose the correct answer!

A missed combined oral contraceptive pill is one that is taken over 24 hours since the time it should have been taken. Missing two or more pills can affect the effectiveness of the contraception and an extra method of contraception will need to be taken for the next seven days.

The need for emergency contraception is determined by which week the pills were missed in and whether sexual intercourse has taken place in the last seven days. Seven days of consecutive pills are thought to be needed to inhibit ovulation – therefore, if the missed pills take place in the first week, emergency contraception will need to be taken (as seven full days of pills will not have been taken). Here, the missed pills are in the second week and therefore, emergency contraception is not required.

If the missed pills occur in the third and final week, two packs are advised to be run together (i.e. no pill-free week should occur).

ANSWERS

93 **Answer**: C – Administer the next injection, offer emergency contraception, additional contraception or abstinence should be advised for the next seven days and a pregnancy test should be carried out in 21 days.

*Explanation*: The DMPA (Depo-Provera) injection is usually administered every 12 weeks and contains progesterone as a long-acting reversible contraceptive (LARC).

However, it is thought that the injection will be effective for up to 14 weeks between injections in most individuals. Overdue is therefore counted as 14 weeks + 1 day.

As sexual intercourse has occurred within the last three days and the woman is overdue her injection, a repeat injection could be administered and emergency contraception should be offered (either copper IUD or progesterone-only emergency contraception), with the advice of additional contraception for the next seven days and a pregnancy test 21 days later. If sexual intercourse had occurred more than five days previously, the woman should not be offered the injection (as there is a risk of pregnancy) and would also be outside the timeframe where emergency contraception could be offered.

# HEAVY MENSTRUAL BLEEDING

*Source*: NICE Clinical Guidline 44: Heavy menstrual bleeding (January 2007)

94 **Answer**: B – Uterine artery embolisation

*Explanation*: Fibroids can be a huge problem for women, causing heavy menstrual bleeding, pressure pain and even subfertility. Treatments such as the levonorgestrel IUS will simply not improve symptoms in these women and of course, not help with subfertility problems.

Uterine artery embolisation (UAE) is fast becoming a method of choice in certain centres where women wish to retain fertility and indeed manage fibroids in order to potentially improve fertility. NICE state that within the UK registry of patients who have undergone the procedure, the vast majority of patients have improved symptoms both at 6 months and at 24 months (84% and 83% respectively).

There have been many case reports of pregnancies following UAE. NICE report a 50% conception rate compared to 78% with myomectomy from one randomised controlled trial.

95 **Answer**: E – Myomectomy

*Explanation*: Whilst more and more women are choosing UAE as a method to retain fertility (see above), it remains that the best and most evidence for any procedure retaining fertility has to be myomectomy.

NICE report a 48% live birth rate (compared to 19% for UAE) from a randomised controlled trial, with a 23% miscarriage rate.

96 **Answer**: H – GnRH analogues for three months prior to hysterectomy

*Explanation*: Whilst hysterectomy would not be considered a first-line treatment, this is still an option in an appropriate situation where the woman is fully informed.

Ideally, GnRH analogues should be administered to shrink the size of the fibroids prior to surgery to reduce the complication rate and assist with the technical difficulty of the surgery.

# CONTRACEPTION PROBLEMS

*Source*: Faculty of Sexual and Reproductive Healthcare:
Management of unscheduled bleeding in women using hormonal
contraception (May 2009); Faculty of Sexual and Reproductive
Healthcare: Contraception for women aged over 40 years
(July 2010)

97 **Answer**: B – Take a full sexual history and commence a
30 mcg or 35 mcg COCP. If not resolving, consider
endometrial biopsy.

*Explanation*: Unscheduled bleeding is bleeding that is not
expected when using hormonal contraception and it can be
classified into various types, including irregular, frequent,
prolonged, etc.

The basic premise for assessing women with unscheduled
bleeding is to take a full history, exclude risks of sexually
transmitted infections, assess risk of pregnancy and take a
cervical smear history.

Unscheduled bleeding is common within the first three
months of starting a new hormonal contraception and if there
are no risk factors for a sexually transmitted infection or cervical
problem, then pelvic examination may not be necessary.

Generally, perseverance for three months may resolve the
problem, or a higher dose of oestrogen may help. As her age
and polycystic ovarian syndrome puts her at risk of endometrial carcinoma, an endometrial biopsy may be required.

98 **Answer**: C – Take a full sexual history and investigate
for STIs if appropriate

*Explanation*: As the patient's irregular bleeding has been
going on for longer than three months and she is in a new

relationship, careful attention should be paid to her sexual history and the risk of any sexually transmitted infection that could be a cause of the irregular bleeding. Her age is also another risk factor for an STI.

99 **Answer**: A – Leave in for a further 12 months and then remove or check two FSH levels, six weeks apart, and if both over 30 IU/L, remove.

*Explanation*: Whilst there is a natural decline in fertility after the mid-30s, pregnancy is still possible and therefore, women should be encouraged to use contraception where this is not wanted. If the levonorgestrel IUS is inserted at or after the age of 45, it can left for seven years or until the woman has gone through the menopause. This can be difficult to detect if the woman is amenorrheic, which commonly occurs after the first year of use.

If the woman is not amenorrheic, any abnormal bleeding patterns should be investigated and contraception should be continued for one year of amenorrhoea after the age of 55.

100 **Answer**: G – Remove the device now

Usually copper coils or IUDs (intrauterine devices) are licensed for five years' use or longer, many for 10 years' use. After a year of amenorrhoea in a woman aged over 45 using non-hormonal contraception, the chances of menstruation and therefore, ovulation, are minimal (World Health Organization state 2–10%).

Therefore, women can be advised to stop using the copper IUD after one year of amenorrhoea if aged over 50. There is no need for routine FSH levels as with hormonal contraception.

# COLPOSCOPY AND CERVICAL SMEARS

*Source*: Colposcopy and Programme Management: Guidelines for the NHS Cervical Screening Programme, second edition (May 2010)

The aim of cervical screening is to look for pre-cancerous changes on the cervix, which can be treated to prevent progression to cervical cancer. These scenarios tended to ask more about special circumstances where it is required that you know the guidelines in detail.

101  **Answer**: E – Repeat smear 3–4 months postnatally

*Explanation*: As the cervix undergoes change during pregnancy, undertaking colposcopy during pregnancy needs a high level of expertise. As mild dyskaryosis may indeed regress of its own accord and not develop into high-grade pathology, most women with low-grade pathology, even outside of pregnancy, would not be treated at the first smear showing evidence of mild dyskaryosis, as CIN I does not necessarily require treatment. Therefore, the repeat smear can be left until 3–4 months postnatally.

102  **Answer**: F – Refer for urgent colposcopy

*Explanation*: All women who have renal failure requiring dialysis should have a cervical smear performed at the time of or shortly after diagnosis. These women have a higher risk of CIN and indeed, cervical cancer. Because of this, any cytological abnormality should be referred for urgent colposcopy. There is some research evidence that in these situations, cytology is insensitive and any co-existing CIN may not be picked up.

**ANSWERS**

## 103 **Answer**: I – Repeat smear in 12 months

*Explanation*: HIV-positive women should have annual screening as HPV can co-exist. However, the use of HAART (highly active anti-retroviral therapy) may also reduce the HPV viral load and therefore, reduce the chance of cervical abnormality. High-grade lesions are managed in the same way as in the HIV negative population, as too are low-grade lesions, which may just represent persistent HPV infection and regress spontaneously.

# MANAGEMENT OF CERVICAL CARCINOMA

*Source*: Colposcopy and Programme Management: Guidelines for the NHS Cervical Screening Programme, second edition (May 2010)

104  **Answer**: F – Trachelectomy

*Explanation*: Stage 1B1 – the cancer can only be seen by a microscope; >5 mm deep and >7 mm wide; if can be seen without a microscope the lesion must be 4 cm or smaller. Trachelectomy as a fertility sparing surgery might be suitable in this situation after appropriate counselling.

105  **Answer**: M – Cone biopsy

*Explanation*: Stage 1A1 – a very small amount of cancer that can only be seen by a microscope and is not more than 3 mm deep and not more than 7 mm wide. Although LLETZ might be enough in this situation, it has to be borne in mind that LLETZ will cause thermal injury to the edges, therefore not providing clear excision margins, and therefore a cone biopsy or even a NETZ is more appropriate. This question has been included to highlight the limitation of LLETZ in cancer.

106  **Answer**: I – See and treat LLETZ

*Explanation*: As colposcopy has confirmed the smear findings, a 'See and treat LLETZ' can be performed, as this would both be diagnostic and therapeutic.

107  **Answer**: E – Postmenopausal bleeding pathway

*Explanation*: Although this looks very much like an advanced cancer, after appropriate resuscitation, tissue diagnosis will be essential before instituting treatment and hence she will need investigation through the PMB pathway.

108 **Answer**: G – Radical surgery with radiotherapy

Stage 1B2 – the cancer can be seen without a microscope and is larger than 4 cm. Definitive surgery is needed in this case.

CIN I, II, III and invasion, and their treatment are very important. Similarly, stage 1 with its subdivisions into A1 and A2 and B1 and B2 are also important. Although there is a move away from radical surgery, this question tries to make sure that this is not missed when necessary.

# RECURRENT MISCARRIAGE

*Source*: RCOG Green Top Guideline No 17: The investigation and treatment of couples with recurrent first-trimester and second-trimester miscarriage (April 2011)

109 **Answer**: B – Referral to geneticist

*Explanation*: This scenario occurs in 2–5% of couples that experience recurrent miscarriage, which is why cytogenetic analysis from the last miscarriage can be insightful. Referral to a geneticist can help as pre-implantation genetic diagnosis may be an option for this couple.

Genetic counselling also offers the couple analysis with regard to the risk of the anomaly occurring again in a subsequent naturally conceived pregnancy.

110 **Answer**: F – Low-dose aspirin and low-molecular-weight heparin

*Explanation*: This woman fits the criteria to be diagnosed with anti-phospolipid syndrome (APS): the presence of anti-phospholipid antibodies in the blood 12 weeks apart, plus one of the following:

- three or more consecutive miscarriages before 10 weeks of gestation
- one or more fetal losses after 10 weeks (where they are morphologically normal)
- one or more preterm births before 34 weeks due to placental disease
- vascular thrombosis (unusual sites may be common).

As one of the mechanisms behind APS is related to thrombosis, meta-analysis has revealed that low-dose aspirin and low-molecular-weight heparin significantly reduces the mis-carriage rate by 54% in these individuals.

111   **Answer**: J – Emotional/psychological support

*Explanation*: Because of the evidence for the answer to question 110, many clinicians have begun to use a combination of aspirin and low-molecular-weight heparin or aspirin alone to help women who have no known explanation for their recurrent miscarriage. However, there is no evidence for this.

The guideline states that 75% of these women have an excellent prognosis for future pregnancy with supportive care alone.

# OUTPATIENT HYSTEROSCOPY: BEST PRACTICE

*Source*: RCOG Green Top Guideline No 59: Best practice in outpatient hysteroscopy (March 2011)

112 **Answer**: B – Use a non-steroidal anti-inflammatory drug one hour before the procedure

*Explanation*: Routine opiate analgesia can cause side-effects and therefore, should be avoided. However, some studies have shown that non-steroidal anti-inflammatories are useful in this situation.

There is limited evidence as to the optimal timing of administration, but one hour before is the guidance recommended by the guideline as the pain relief will be effective by the time of the procedure.

113 **Answer**: C – Offer a chaperone

*Explanation*: It is good practice to always offer a chaperone, even though the doctor is herself female. This is to protect both the patient and the doctor. Documentation of this offer and presence should occur.

114 **Answer**: D – Use normal saline as the distension medium.

*Explanation*: Whilst for investigative hysteroscopy, the distension medium is at the discretion of the operator (as there is little difference in image quality and pain levels for the patient); for all electrosurgical procedures, normal saline should be used as it is required to conduct during the procedure.

# HYSTEROSCOPY AND ENDOMETRIAL PATHOLOGY

*Source*: Cooper N.A.M., Smith P., Khan K.S. and Clark T.J. Vaginoscopic approach to outpatient hysteroscopy: a systematic review of the effect on pain. *British Journal of Obstetrics and Gynaecology* 2010; **117**(5): 532–539.

Tsimpanakos I. *et al.* Vaginoscopic approach to outpatient hysteroscopy: a systematic review of the effect of pain. *British Journal of Obstetrics and Gynaecology* 2010; **117**(9): 1163–1164.

Chin J., Konje J. and Hickey M. Levonorgestrel intrauterine system for endometrial protection in women with breast cancer on adjuvant tamoxifen. *Cochrane Database of Systematic Reviews* 2009 Oct 7; (4): CD007245.

115  **Answer**: B – Perform hysteroscopy +/– polypectomy

*Explanation*: Vaginoscopy does not reduce failure rates in hysteroscopy

116  **Answer**: C – Offer levonorgestrel intrauterine system

*Explanation*: An effective medical form of endometrial protection to avoid surgery

117  **Answer**: A – Perform annual screening for endometrial cancer

*Explanation*: Her risk of endometrial cancer is 30–60%

118  **Answer**: E – Reassure

*Explanation*: The lining of the endometrium is thin.

119 **Answer**: D – Consider changing contraception, if
any; then wait and see

*Explanation*: This may be a side-effect of the progesterone
and therefore, a different contraceptive may very well have a
different effect.

# MANAGEMENT OF VULVAL SKIN DISORDERS

*Source*: RCOG Green Top Guideline No 58: The management of vulval skin disorders (February 2011)

120 **Answer**: B – Clobetasol

*Explanation*: This is an example of lichen sclerosus. It is an autoimmune disorder and can be associated with diabetes, hypothyroidism and/or premature ovarian failure. There is significant morbidity associated with this condition. Treatment with clobetasol is the appropriate management.

121 **Answer**: I – General measures

*Explanation*: Chronic vulval dermatosis or lichen simplex chronic – treatment here is with general measures and emollients.

122 **Answer**: C – Immunomodulators

*Explanation*: Recurrent oral and genital ulcers are manifestations of Behcet's disease/syndrome. Treatment is with steroids, immunosuppressants and immunomodulators (C or L). If the problem is long term, it might be more appropriate to consider immunomodulators (C).

123 **Answer**: F – Local excision

*Explanation*: This is a classic example of the usual type of VIN with warty plaque-like lesions. It is associated with chronic immunosuppression, smoking, HPV infection and intraepithelial neoplasia. Although anti-histamines, emollients etc. are used for symptom relief, the treatment of choice is wide local excision.

124 **Answer**: B – Clobetasol

*Explanation*: Vulval psoriasis affects the vulva, but not the vaginal mucosa. They are characterised by discrete lesions and are different from lesions in the non-genital sites. Emollients, soap substitutes, steroids, calcipotrients are generally used for treatment; however, coal tar should be avoided in the genital area.

125 **Answer**: C – Immunomodulators

*Explanation*: This is a case of advanced inflammatory bowel disease, which can also present with swelling and ulceration on the vulva. Surgical excision is not appropriate.

# TEACHING METHODS

*Source*: Duthie S.J. and Garden A.S. The teacher, the learner and the method. *The Obstetrician and Gynaecologist* 2010; **12**: 273–280.

126 **Answer**: C – Problem-based learning

*Explanation*: Problem-based learning has been used in many UK medical schools as an adult style of learning to encourage medical students from day one to think on their feet and brainstorm problems. There is an onus on the students to be self-directed, with minimal facilitation from the tutor.

127 **Answer**: F – Schema refinement

*Explanation*: In this example, the tutor activates previous knowledge on the subject of PCOS (schema activation) and builds upon that knowledge with illustrated examples (schema refinement).

128 **Answer**: E – Complex procedural hierarchy

*Explanation*: This style of teaching/learning develops over a significant period of time with several different levels of learning. It may also involve more than one tutor. This technique is widely used in the UK when learning surgical procedures such as caesarean section.

129 **Answer**: G – Snowballing

*Explanation*: This technique is commonly used by tutors without even realising it – assessing the level of knowledge of the trainees allows the tutor to know at what level to pitch their tutorial and how to advance their knowledge.

# CAPACITY AND THE MENTAL HEALTH ACT

*Source*: Nicholas N. and Nicholas S. Understanding the Mental Capacity Act 2005: a guide for clinicians. *The Obstetrician and Gynaecologist* 2011; **12**: 29–34.

130 **Answer**: A – Advance directive

*Explanation*: Advance decisions can be made by anyone over the age of 18 about their medical treatment. They must be deemed to have capacity to make this decision – understand the relevant information given to them, retain the information, weigh up the pros and cons, and communicate the decision.

An advance directive documents specific decisions that have been discussed in advance in detail and signed by the maker of the document and a witness.

131 **Answer**: E – Lasting power of attorney

*Explanation*: A person (donor) may appoint another person (donee) to make decisions on their behalf if they lose capacity to make decisions themselves. The donor must be aged over 18, have capacity at the time of appointing the person and also register their authority.

132 **Answer**: H – Consult relevant persons to determine the best interests of the patient

*Explanation*: Doctors are sometimes placed in situations dealing with unconscious patients or with patients who lack capacity or who cannot express their decisions. It is in these situations that we look to relevant persons, such as close family, to help with decision-making. However, the final responsibility lies with the decision-maker.

# PROVIDING INFORMATION ABOUT RISK

*Source*: Consent advice series: Individual consent information procedures on the RCOG website – www.rcog.org.uk

133 **Answer**: D – Uncommon (1/100–1/1000)

*Explanation*: The risk of bladder/ureteric injury during a total abdominal hysterectomy with no additional risk factors is quoted as 7/1000.

134 **Answer**: E – Rare (1/1000–1/10 000)

*Explanation*: Maternal risks are increased during an emergency caesarean section as compared to an elective. However, bladder injury is quoted as 1/1000 and ureteric injury as 3/10 000 (both rare).

135 **Answer**: E – Rare (1/1000–1/10 000)

*Explanation*: Severe sepsis has been reported, but is a rare complication, quoted as less than 1/1000.

# DECISION-MAKING AT SURGERY

*Source*: RCOG Clinical Governance Series: Advice No. 6
(December 2008)

136 **Answer**: C – Leave the mass alone, abandon the
procedure and discuss with the patient once she is
awake, including referral for a specialist opinion

*Explanation*: Even though the woman has consented to a
bilateral salpingo-oophorectomy, it is not known what the
nature of this mass is – either benign or malignant – and
therefore, the mass should be left alone at the time of surgery
and the procedure abandoned.

Following specialist referral (to determine whether the mass
is malignant), the most appropriate surgical procedure or
other form of management can take place – which may
ultimately lead to the same procedure being carried out as
was first planned if the mass is indeed benign.

137 **Answer**: F – Perform a salpingectomy

*Explanation*: From the description, this is almost certainly an
ectopic pregnancy. This would be considered a threat to the
life of the patient, especially as it is rupturing through the
tube and therefore, should be removed (without prior consent) in order to save the patient's life.

A salpingectomy would be the most appropriate procedure
in this scenario.

## ASSESSMENT AND FEEDBACK

*Source*: Shehmar M. and Khan K. A guide to the ATSM in Medical Education. Article 2: assessment, feedback and evaluation. *The Obstetrician and Gynaecologist* 2010; **12**: 119–125.

138 **Answer**: C – Summative assessment

*Explanation*: The assessment described is similar to the ARCP (annual review of competence progression) that occurs in the training system in the UK. It is an end of year assessment, which has a pass/fail element to decide on progression to the next year of training.

139 **Answer**: H – Feedback

*Explanation*: The supervisor here is making a judgement on the trainee's performance, but providing him or her with helpful hints and comments which lead to continuous improvement on their performance.

Don't be confused by the word 'evaluation' or 'appraisal'. In this context, 'evaluation' would mean feedback on a training programme or trainer.

140 **Answer**: D – Evaluation

*Explanation*: As highlighted above, evaluation tends to mean feedback on a training programme or particular trainer, and is usually completed in written form.

# STATISTICS

141 **Answer**: J – 1.62

*Explanation*: RR = risk of br. Ca. in smoker/risk of br. Ca. in non-smoker

= (34/55) / (21/55) = 1.6191 ... = 1.62 to two decimal places.

142 **Answer**: M – 0.03

*Explanation*: To be significant at the 5% level, $p$ has to be *less than* 0.05. Therefore the only possible answer is M.

143 **Answer**: H – Incidence

*Explanation*: 21/1000 = 2.1% ('approx. 2%'). This describes the *incidence* of pregnancies affected.

144 and 145: Approach the problem with a 2 × 2 table for epidemiological study of a disease.

| | | Outcome | | |
|---|---|---|---|---|
| Test Result | Positive | Positive | Negative | |
| | | True positive | False positive | Test positive |
| | Negative | False negative | True negative | Test negative |
| | | Outcome positive | Outcome negative | Total |

Inserting figures into the table we get:

| | | Outcome | | |
|---|---|---|---|---|
| Test Result | Positive | Positive | Negative | |
| | | 18 | 24 | 42 |
| | Negative | 3 | 956 | 958 |
| | | 21 | 979 | 1000 |

144 **Answer**: L – The calculation depicts *specificity*: true negative/outcome negative.

145 **Answer**: F – This calculation depicts *negative predictive value*: true negative/test negative.

# SURGERY IMPROVING FERTILITY OUTCOMES AND UNDERSTANDING STATISTICS

*Source*: Suresh Y.N. and Narveker N. Role of surgery to optimise outcome of assisted conception treatments. *The Obstetrician and Gynaecologist* 2013; **15**: 91–98.

The purpose of this question is not just to ask about success rates, but also to assess your understanding of odds ratio and the language of statistics.

146 **Answer**: M – Odds ratio of 4

*Explanation*: This is the odds ratio of success of pregnancy following treatment.

147 **Answer**: A – Twofold increase in success rate

*Explanation*: As stated, a twofold increase in success rate with treatment versus without.

148 **Answer**: D – Conception rate of 35–84%

149 **Answer**: A – Twofold increase in success rate

150 **Answer**: C – Odds ratio of 1.6

# INDEX

Printed in the United States
By Bookmasters

Printed in the United States
By Bookmasters